AF374804

# MY BIG BOOTS

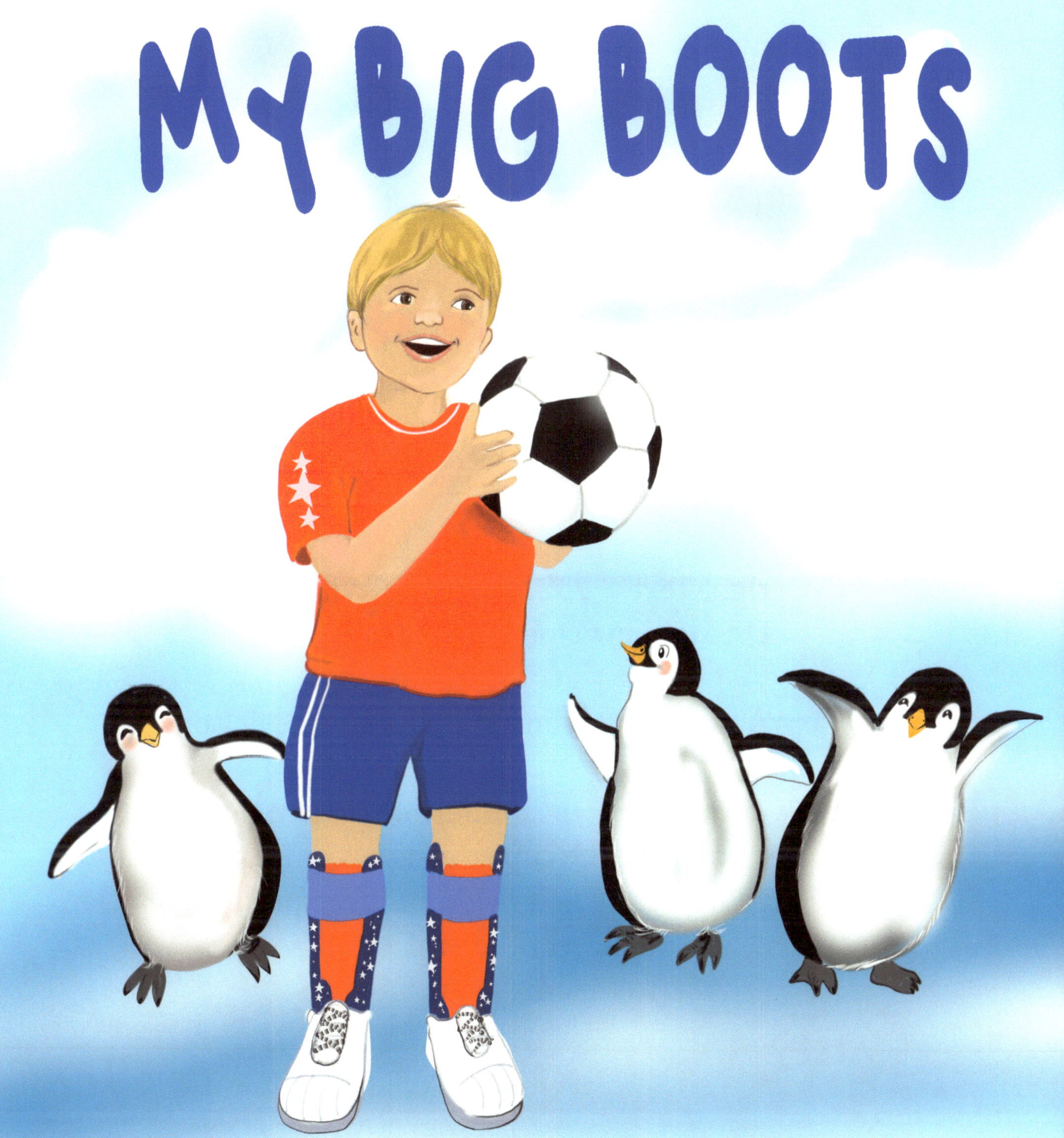

By Dr. Mitzi Williams
with Dr. Matthew Dobbs and Dr. Scott Kaiser
Illustrated by Ginger Nielson

# MY BIG BOOTS

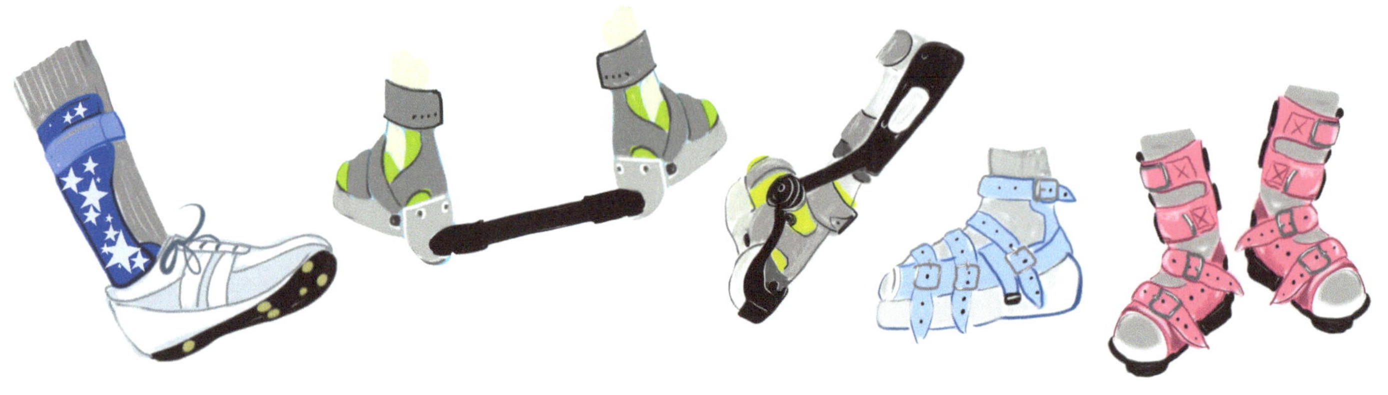

# About the Authors

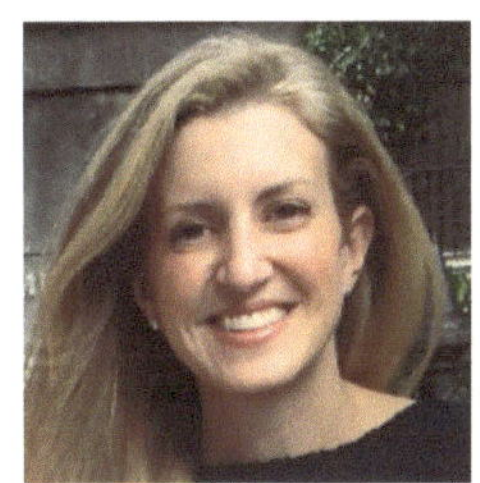

Mitzi Williams DPM, FACFAS is a pediatric foot and lower extremity surgeon who specializes in congenital deformities. Dr. Williams and her colleague, Dr. Scott Kaiser, direct the Pediatric and Infant Foot Deformity Clinic at Kaiser Permanente in Oakland, California. She is an attending surgeon at the SF Bay Area Foot and Ankle Residency Program. Dr. Williams is nationally recognized for her expertise in treating pediatric foot and lower extremity deformities.

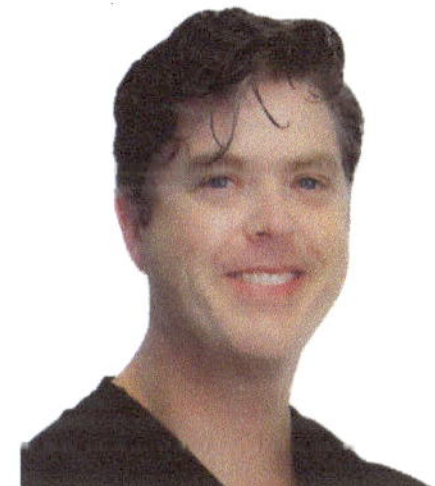

Matthew Dobbs MD, FACS is the director of the Dobbs Clubfoot Center at the Paley Institute in West Palm Beach, Florida. Prior to that, he was the Dr. Asa C. and Mrs. Dorothy W. Jones Professor of Orthopaedic Surgery and the Director of Strategic Planning at Washington University School of Medicine. Dr. Dobbs is internationally recognized for his expertise and innovation in the field of pediatric foot and lower extremity deformities.

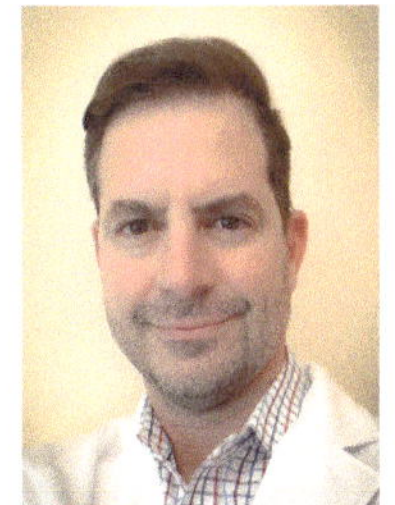

Scott Kaiser MD is a pediatric orthopedic surgeon who specializes in a wide breadth of disorders that affect children's gait. He partners with Dr. Mitzi Williams to direct the Pediatric and Infant Foot Deformity Clinic at Kaiser Permanente in Oakland, California.

We thank our incredible clinical and surgical care teams including Kathy Kreitner, Marissa Bard, Anna Pacheco, and Omar Phillips.

We give special thanks to the patients and their families whose stories inspire us.

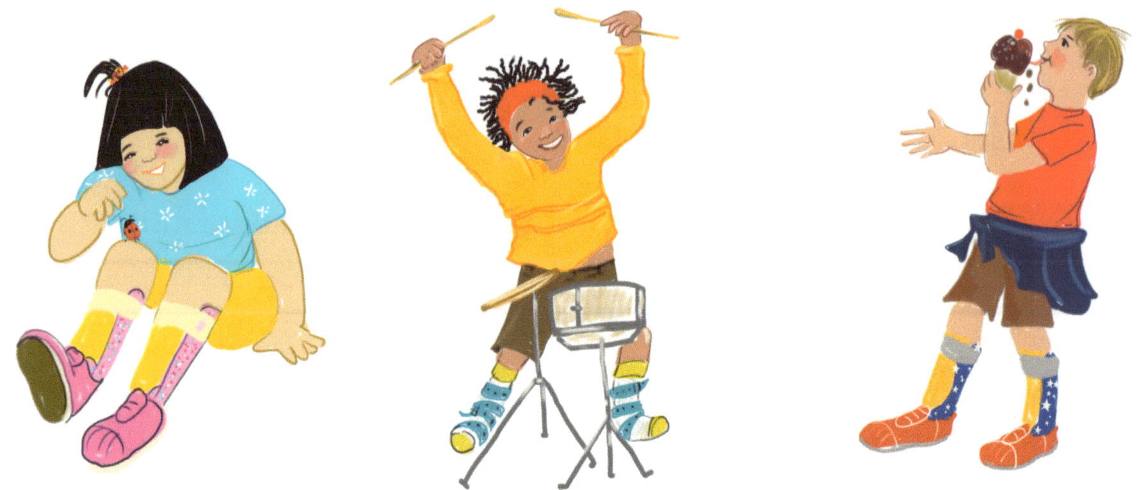

*My Big Boots,* along with its prequel entitled *My Boots,* are dedicated to the children worldwide born with clubfoot. These books share a child's perspective on clubfoot and provide accurate information for their families. We find these books to be helpful tools in  speaking with children about clubfoot. These books are also helpful in aiding in any conversation with siblings and friends of children with clubfoot.

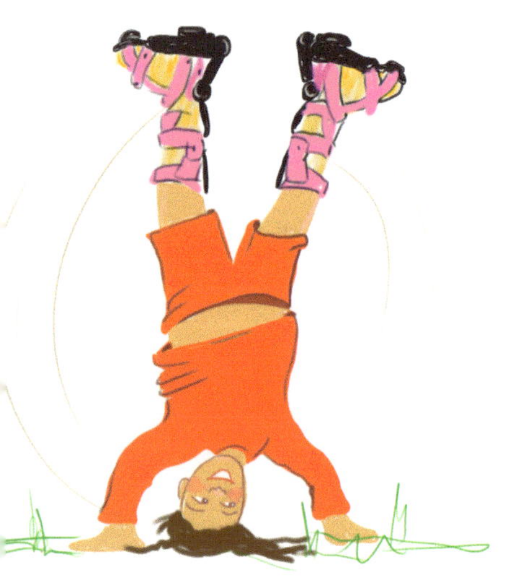

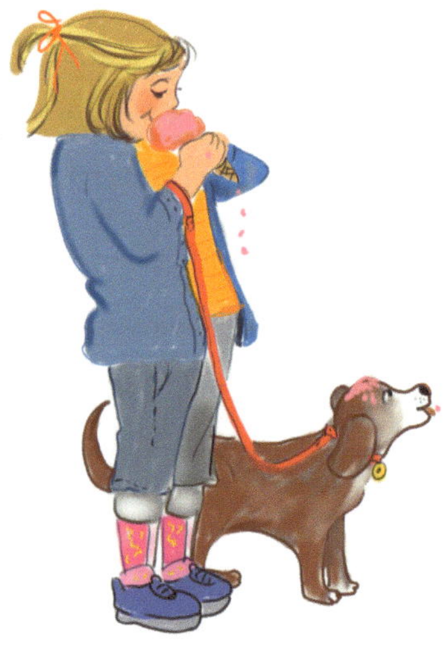

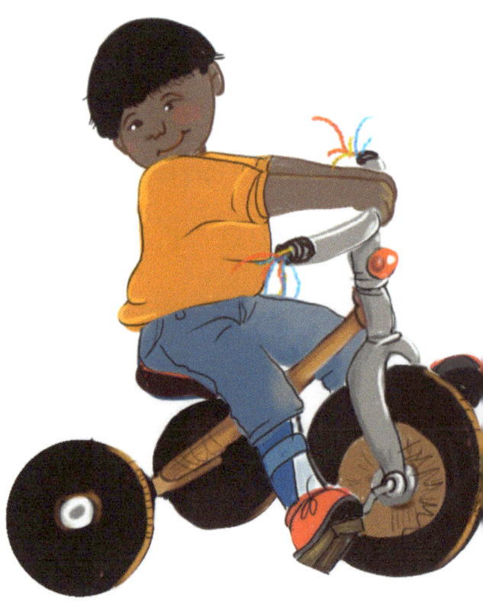

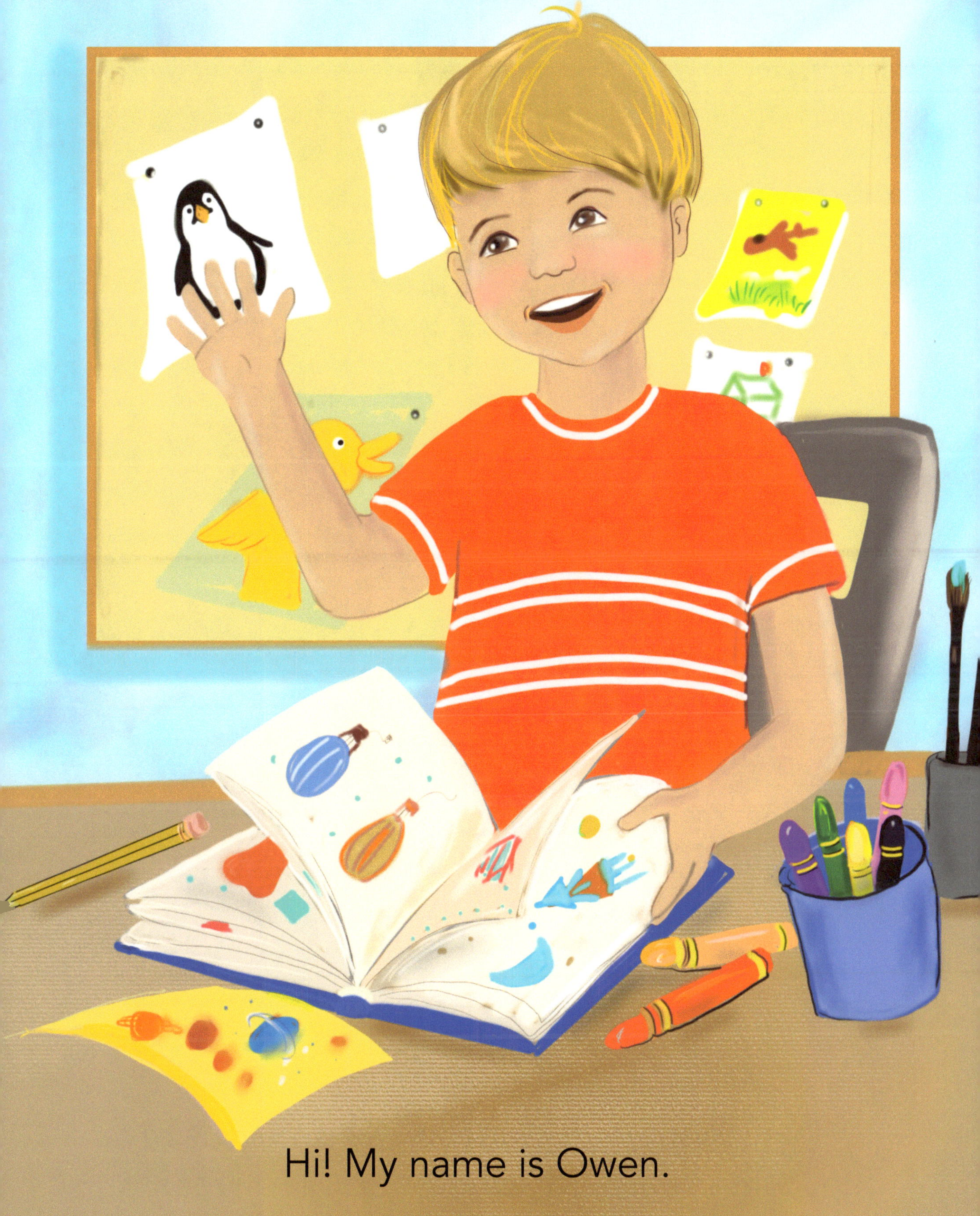

Hi! My name is Owen.

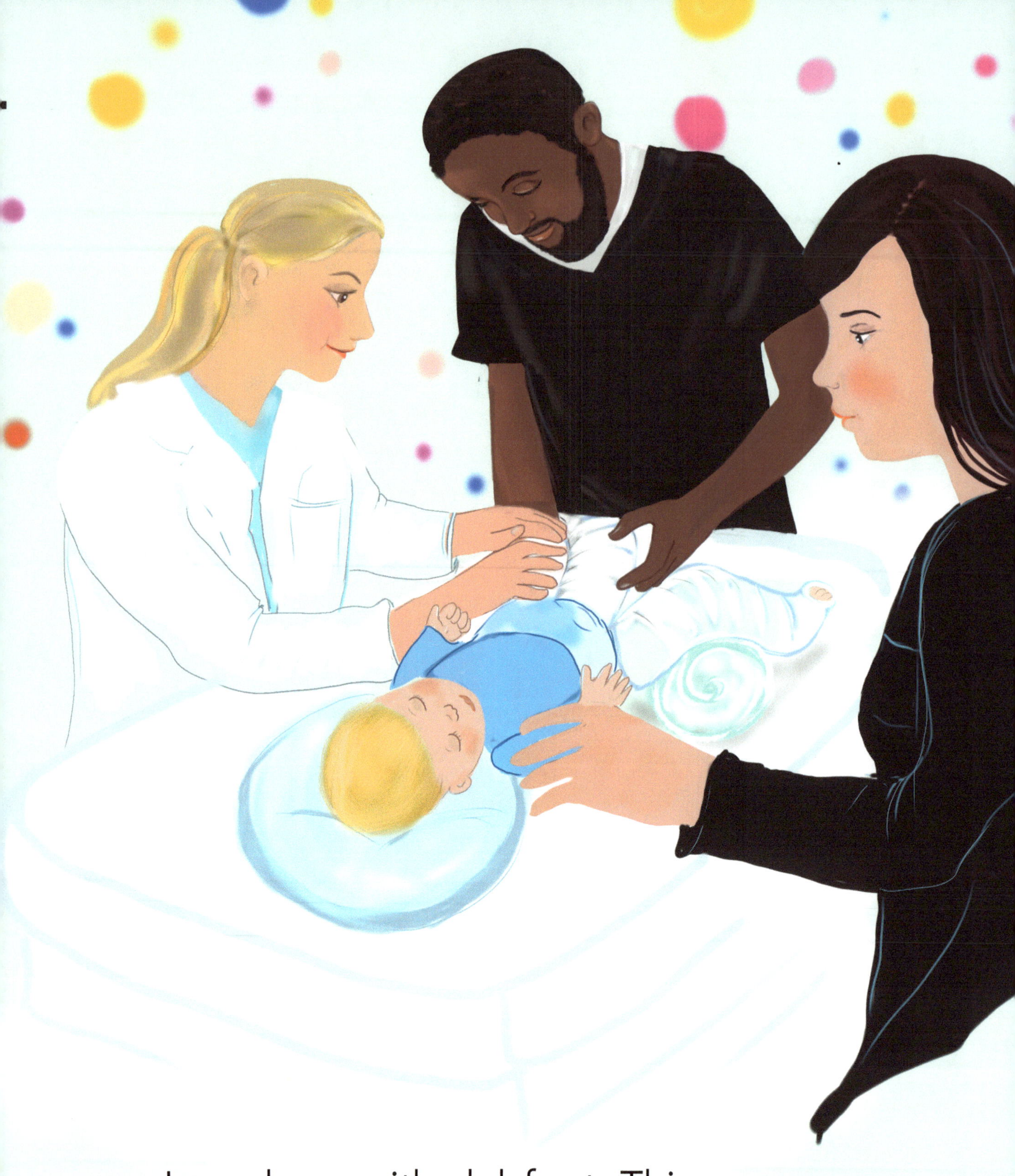

I was born with clubfoot. This means my feet turn inward. My doctor applied weekly casts to help straighten my feet.

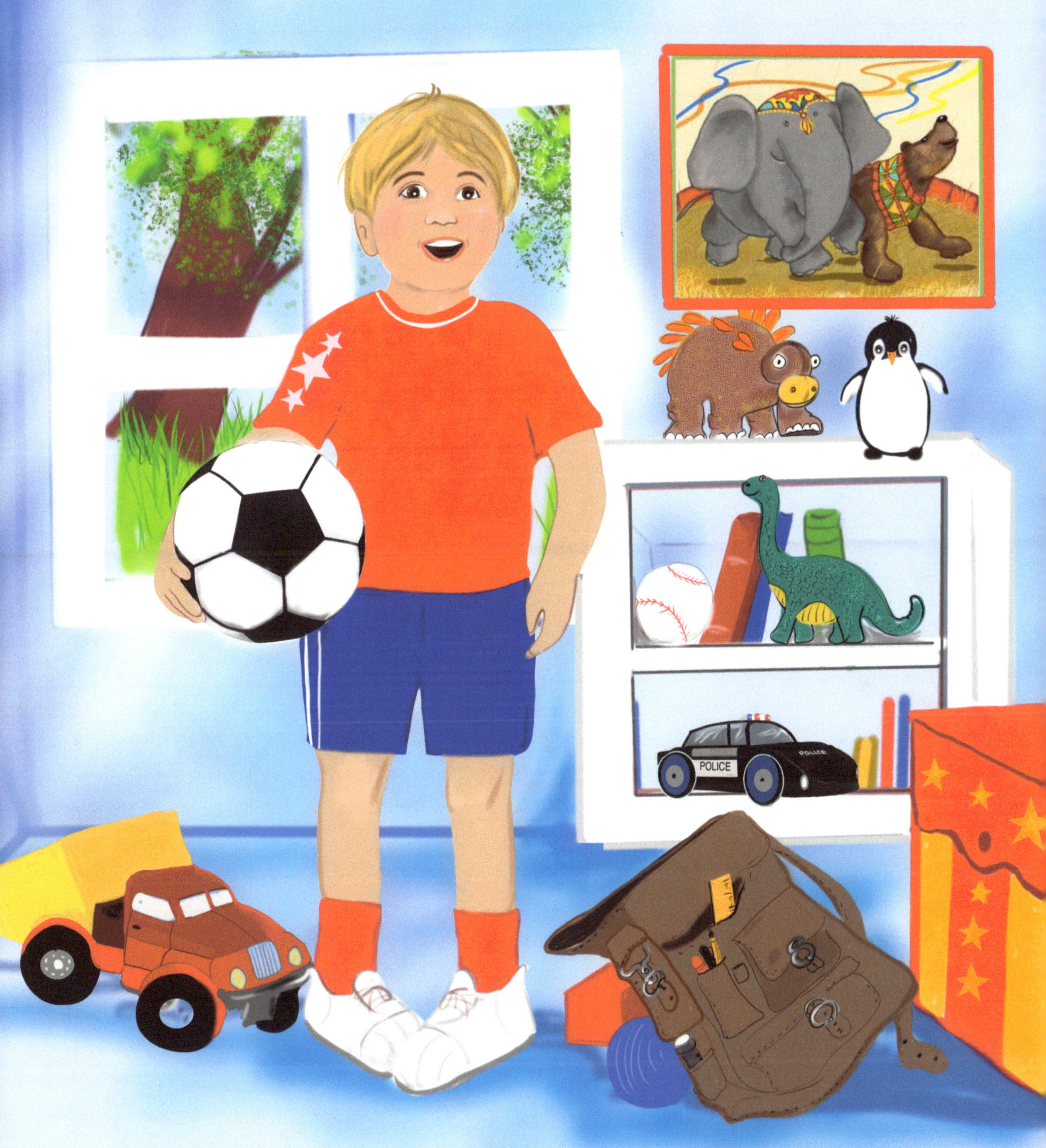

As I grew, my mother noticed that my
feet were turning in again.

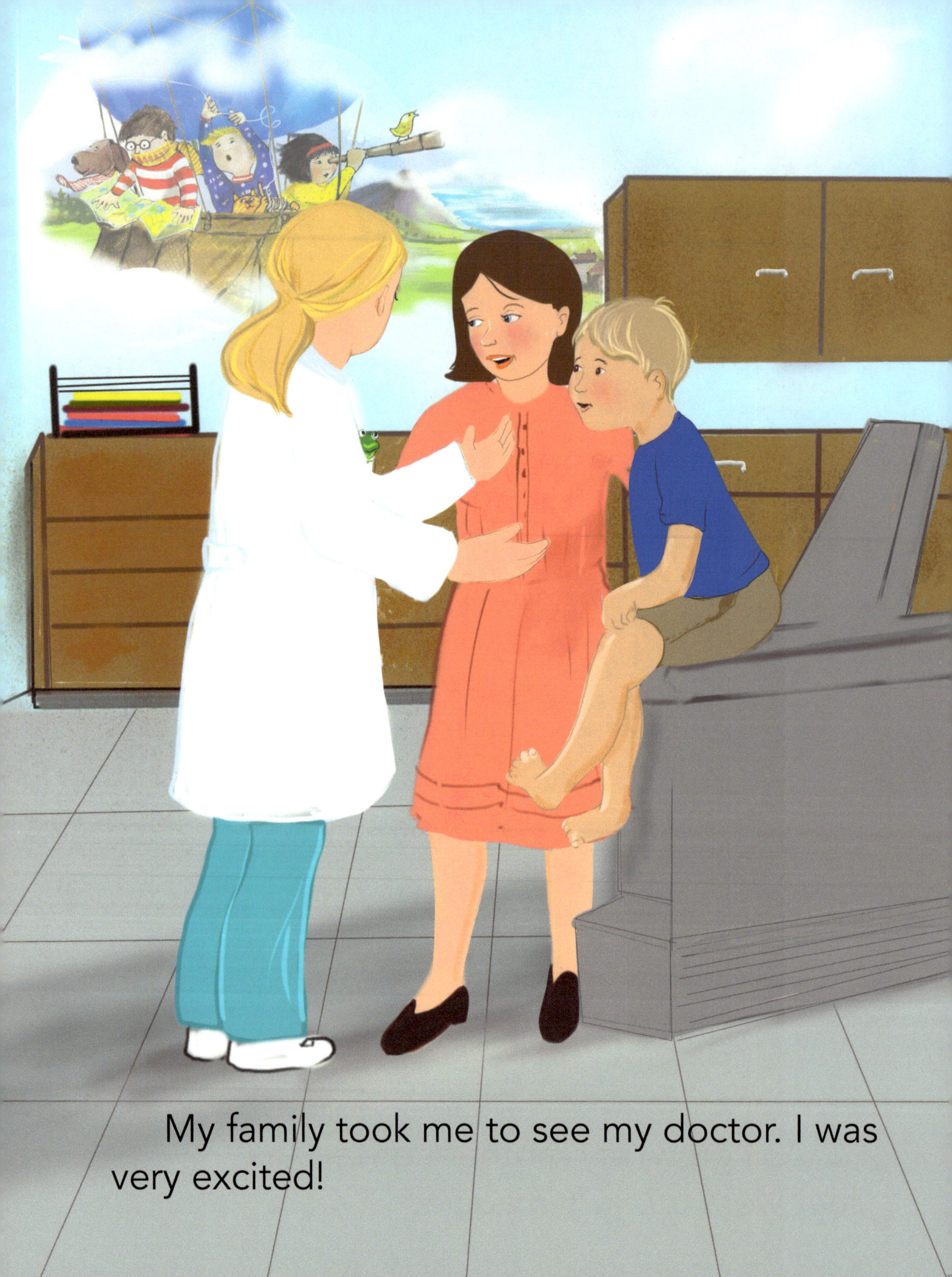

My family took me to see my doctor. I was very excited!

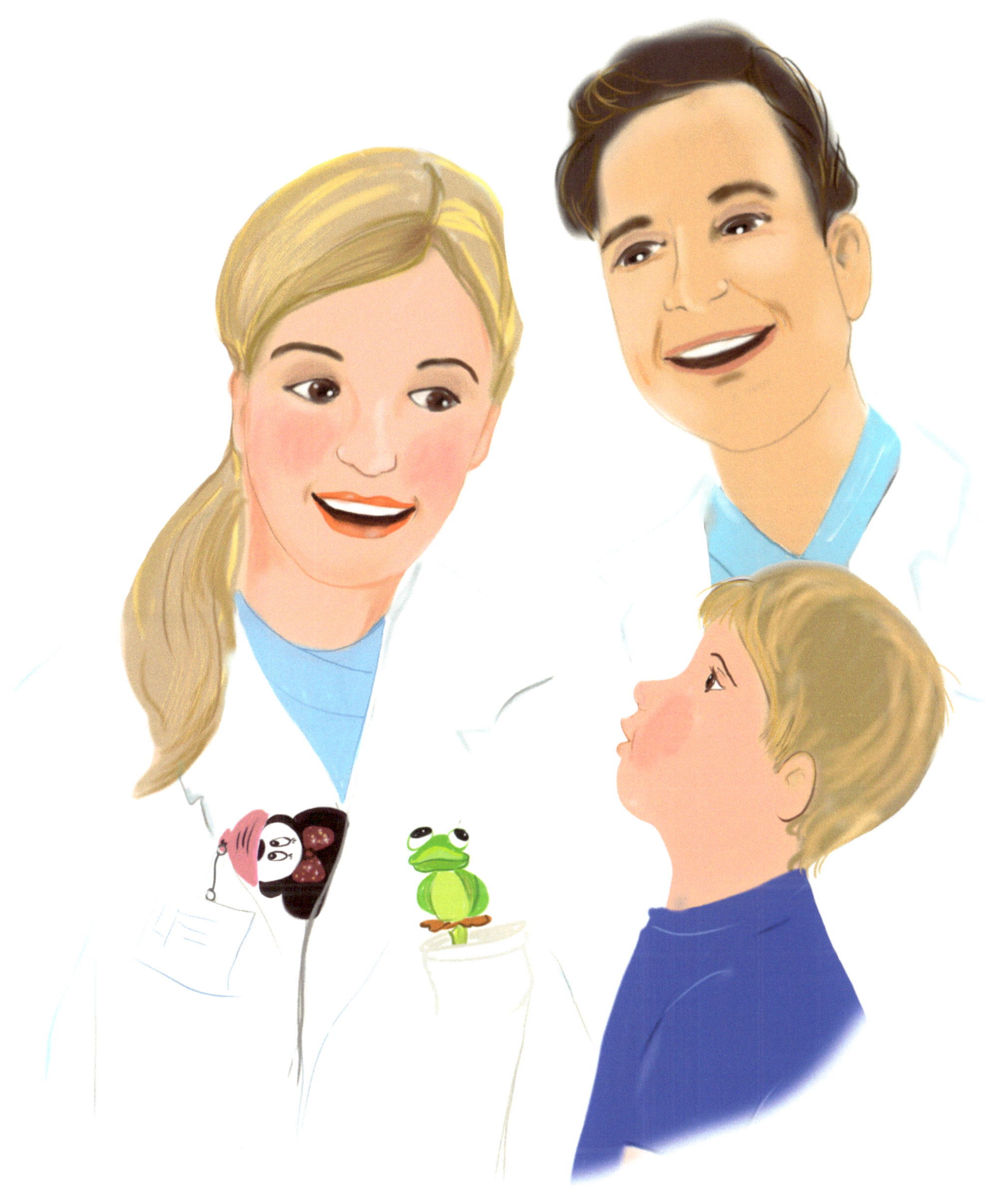

My doctor said clubfoot could recur for many reasons. That means it can come back.

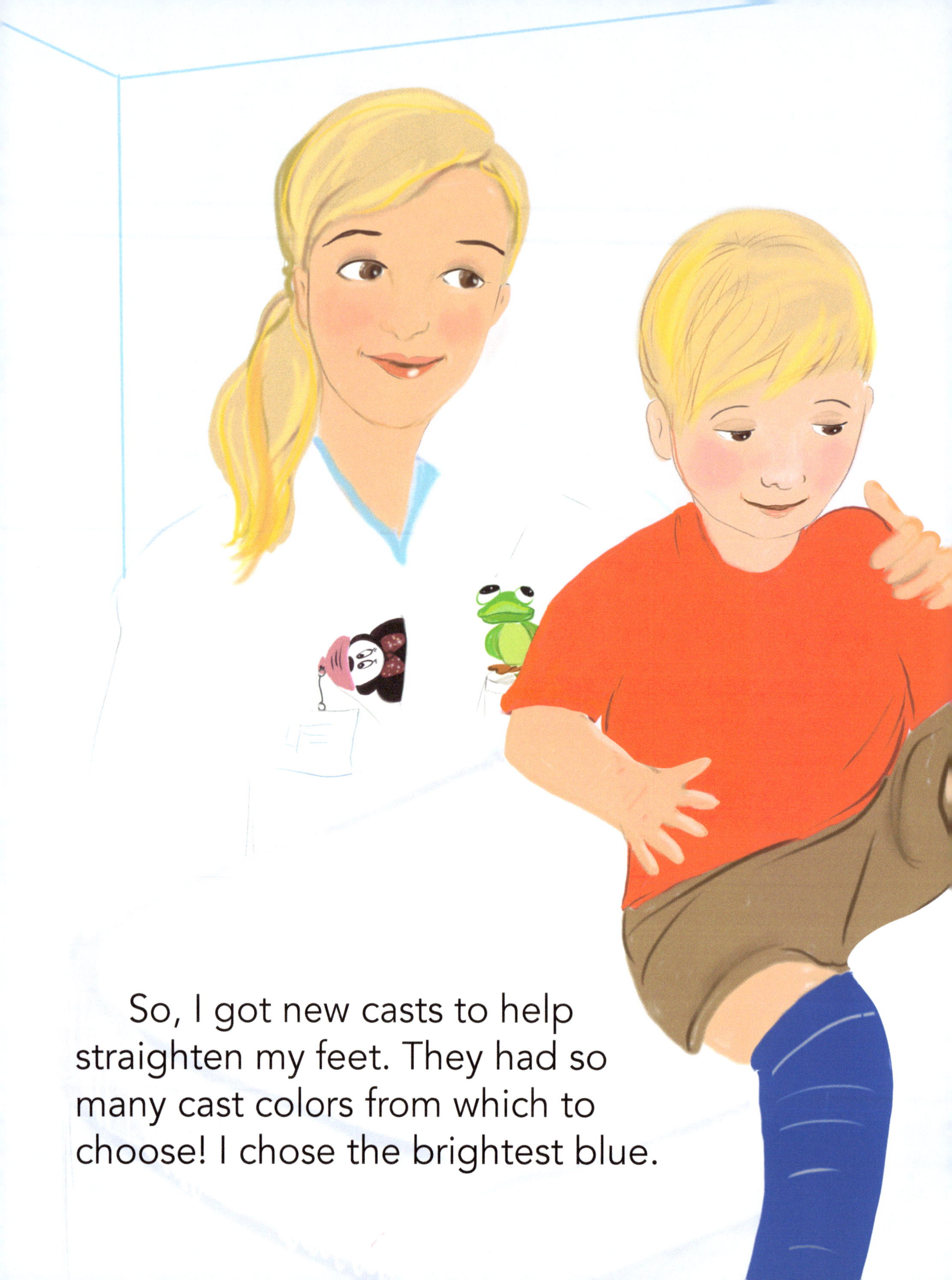

So, I got new casts to help
straighten my feet. They had so
many cast colors from which to
choose! I chose the brightest blue.

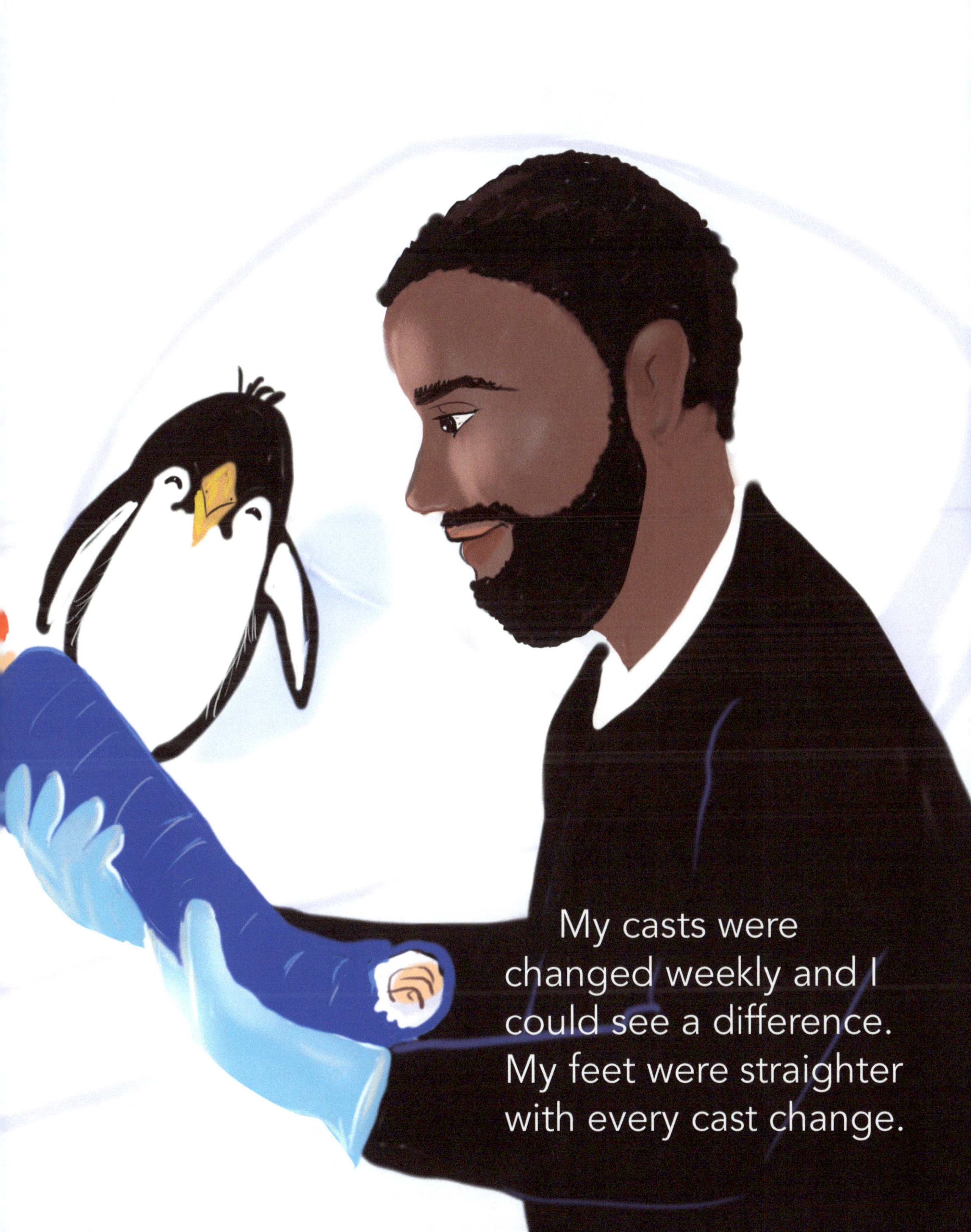

My casts were changed weekly and I could see a difference. My feet were straighter with every cast change.

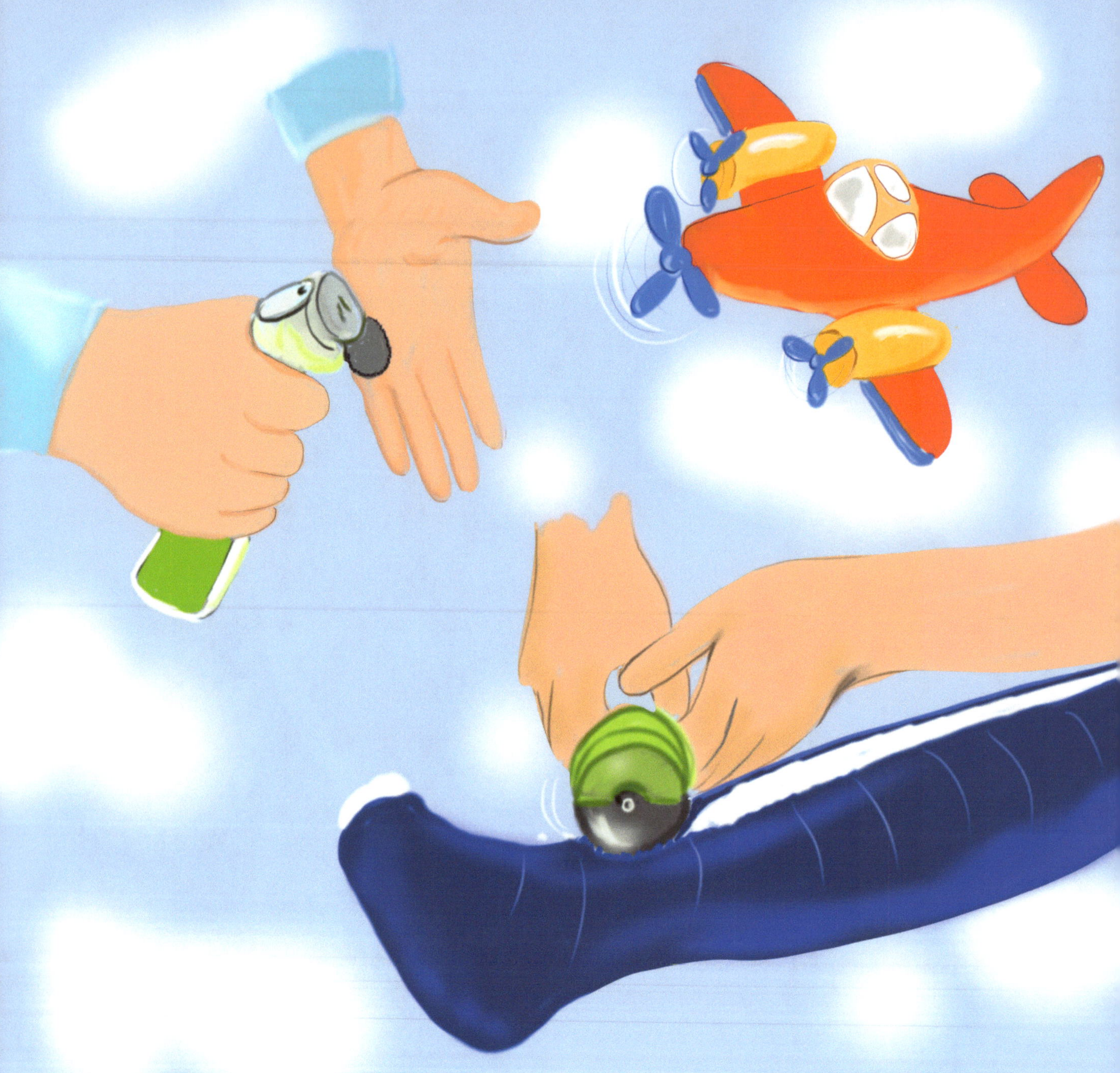

A cast saw was used to remove each cast. It was loud but it did not hurt! The cast saw vibrates so it actually tickled slightly. It sounded like an airplane taking off into the sky!

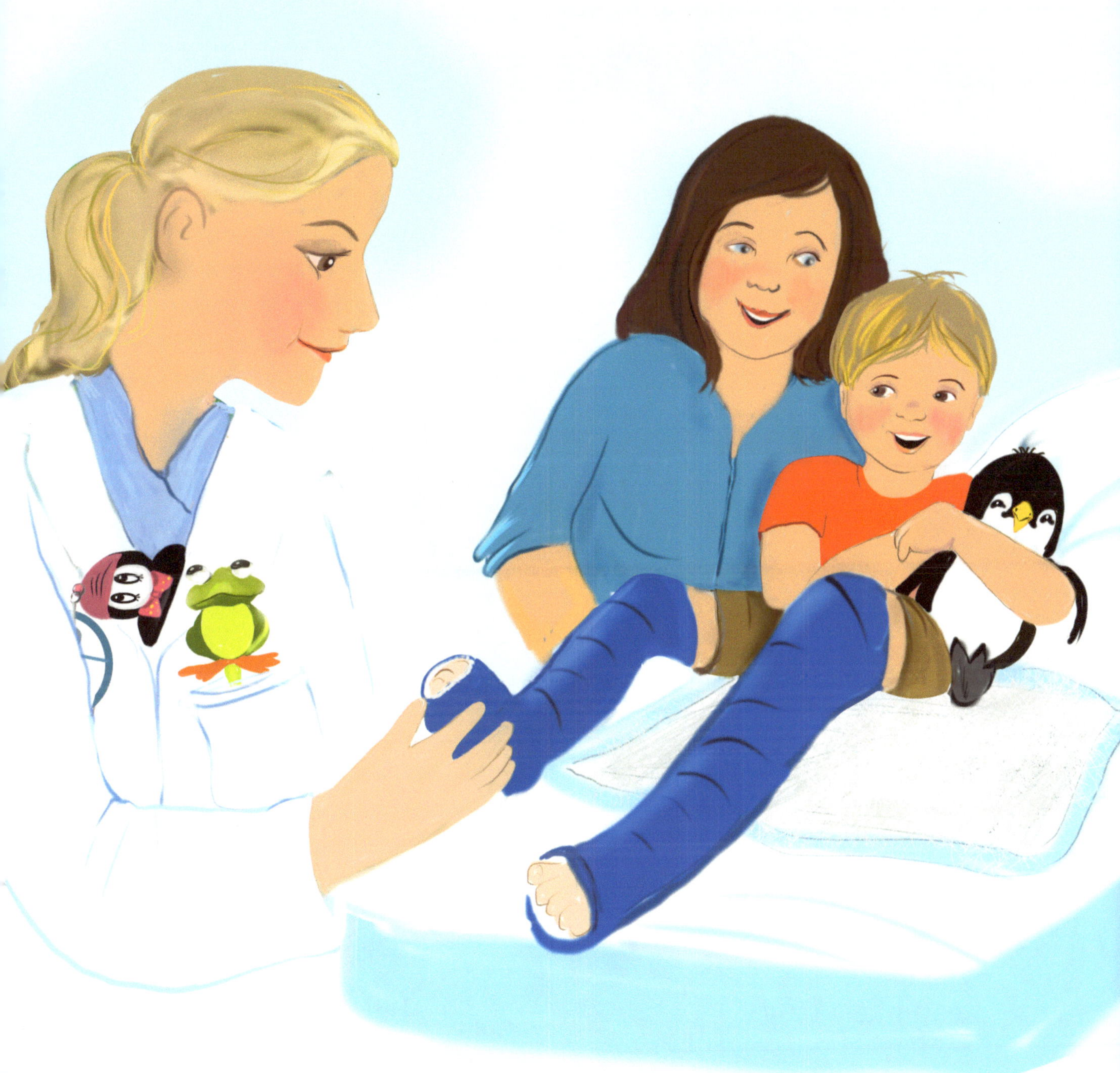

Casting did help straighten my feet while my doctor talked about a surgery that could help my feet even more.

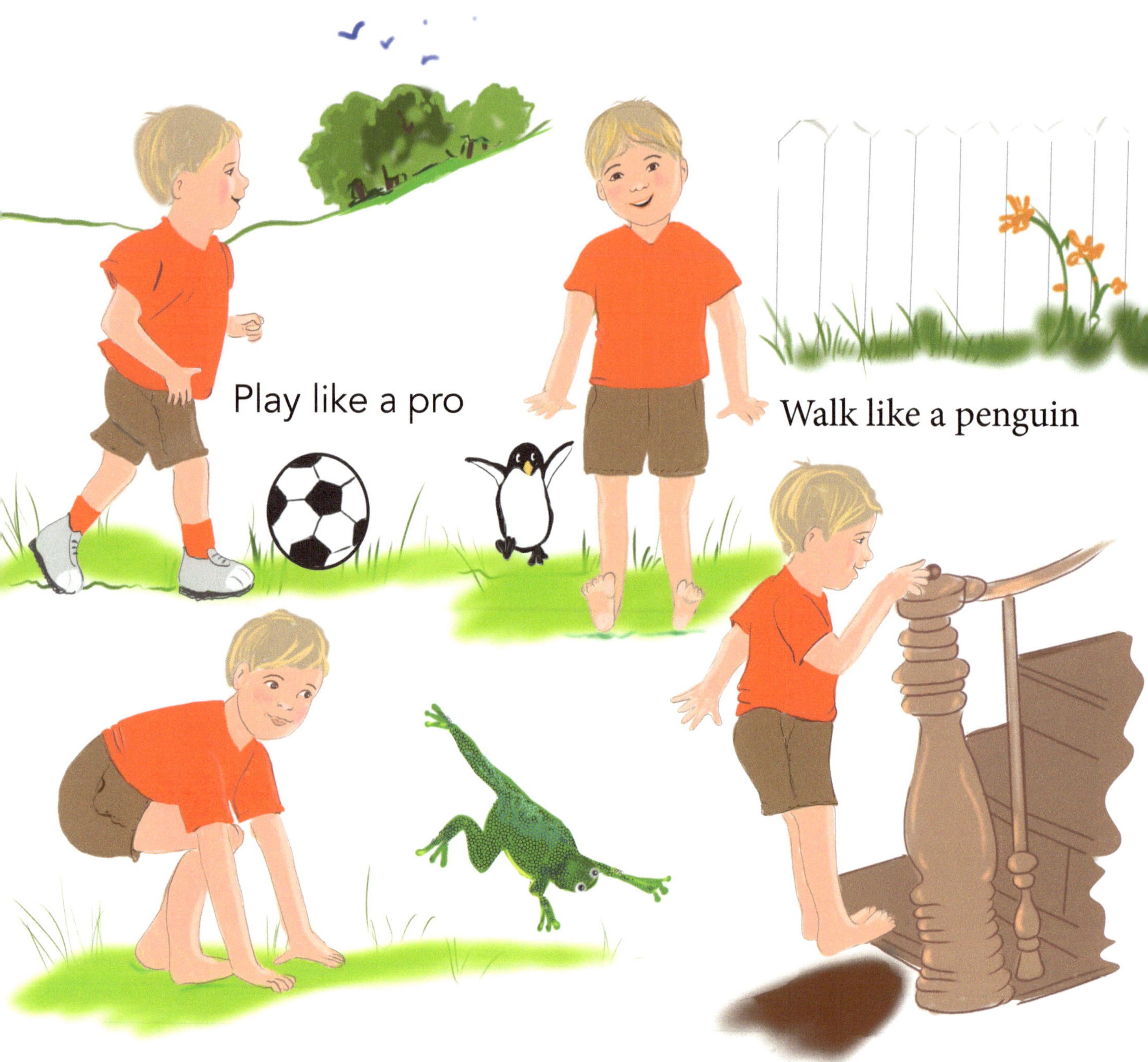


I learned that despite casting or surgery, stretching to keep my feet supple and soft would be helpful. There are many fun activities I can do to stretch my feet.

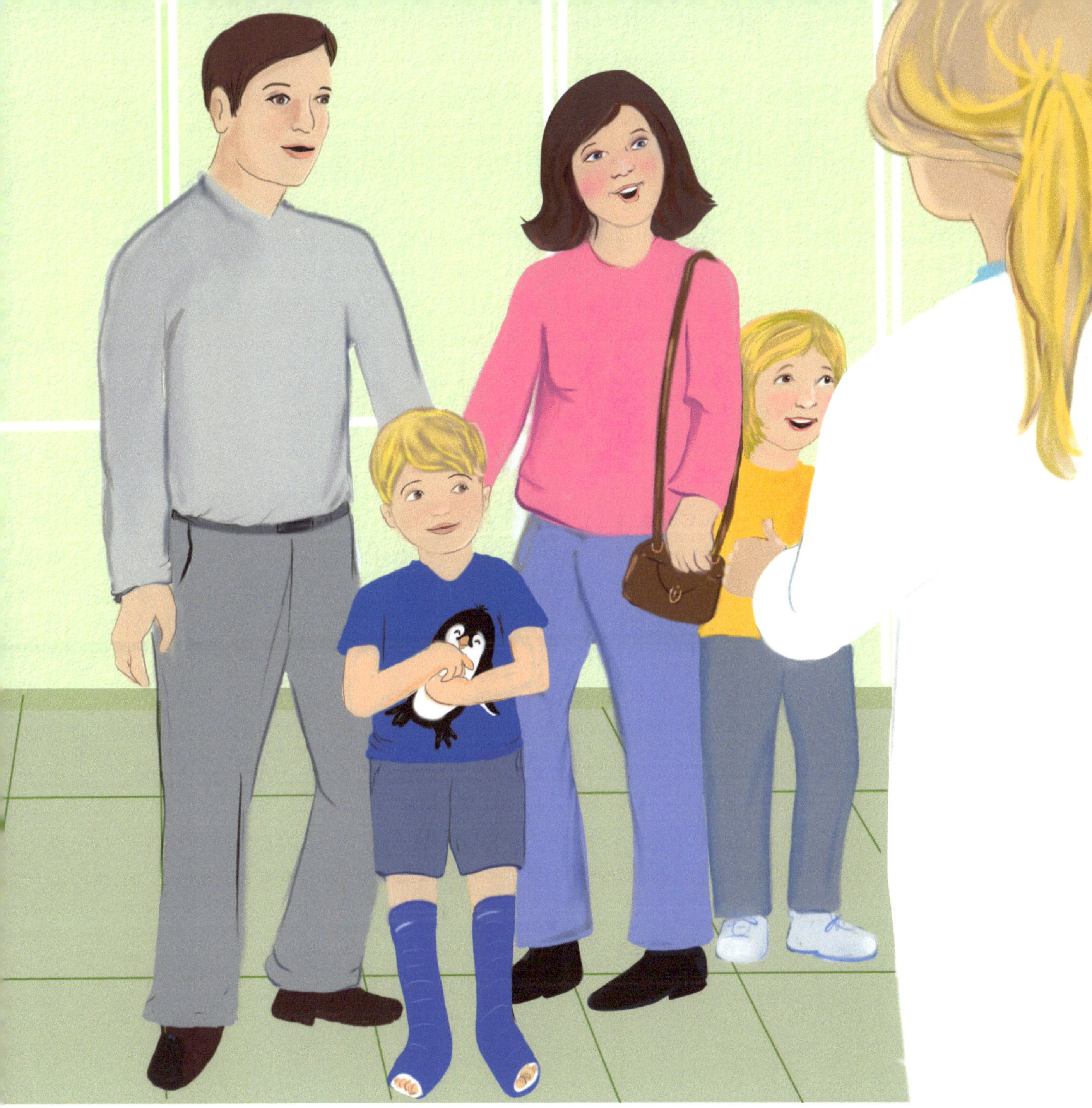

On the day of my surgery, my family awoke very early in the morning to drive to the hospital. My doctor met us there. The nurses and hospital staff were so nice and friendly to me.

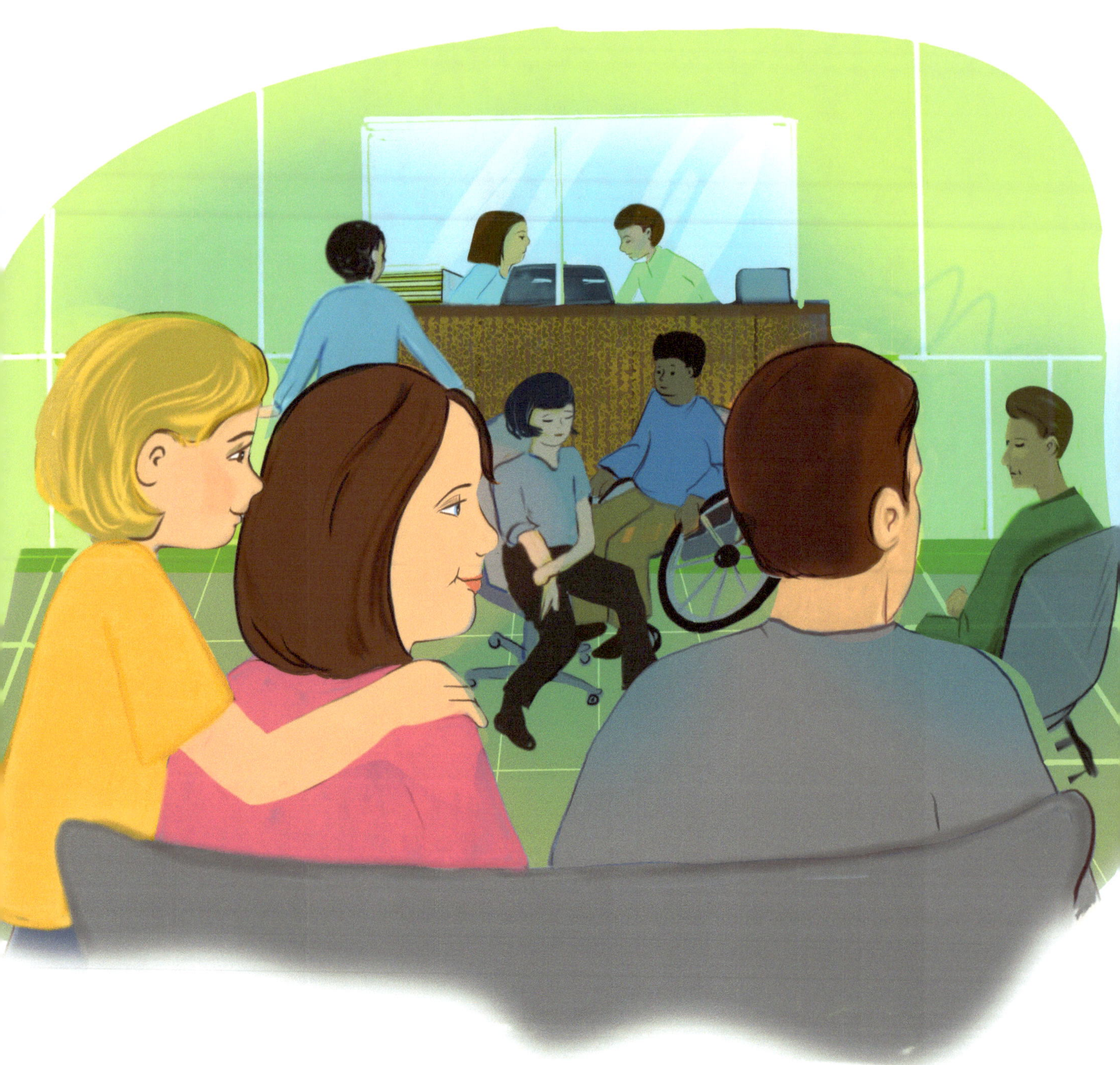

Being in the hospital was a new experience for me. There were so many nice people there to keep me safe and healthy.

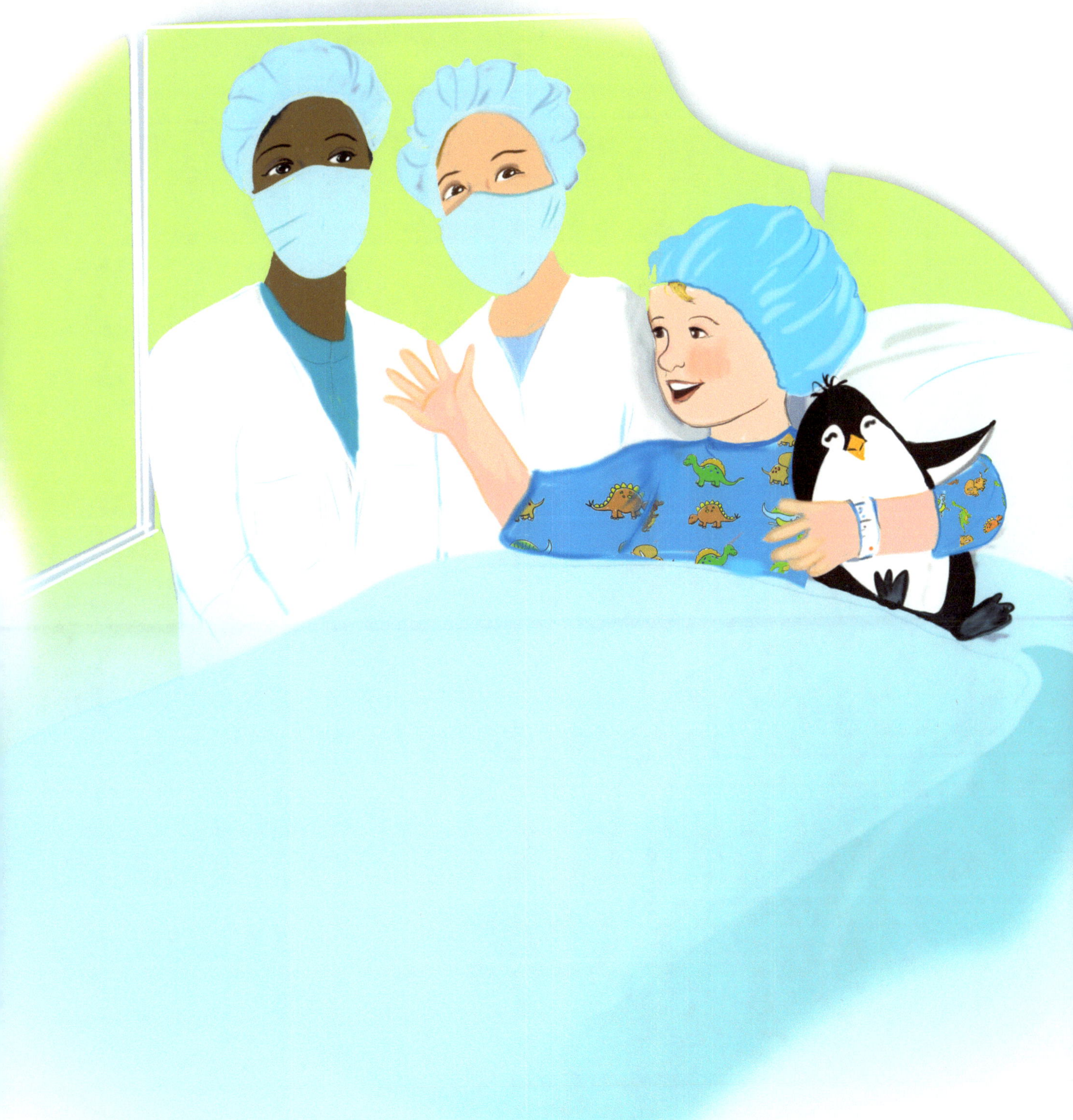

The nurses brought me to the operating room while my family waited in the waiting room for me.

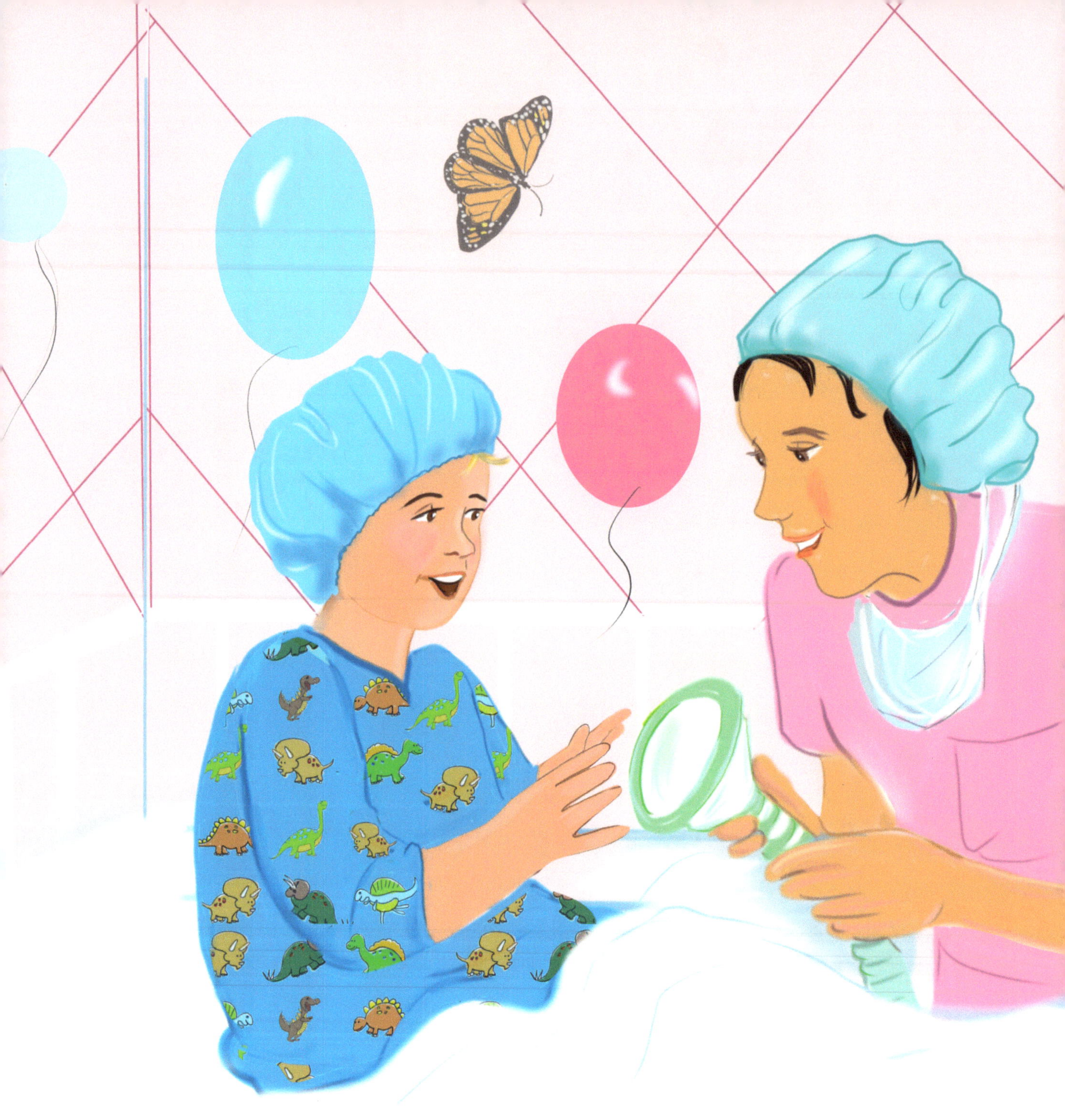

In the operating room, I breathed into  a plastic mask. I smelled strawberry!

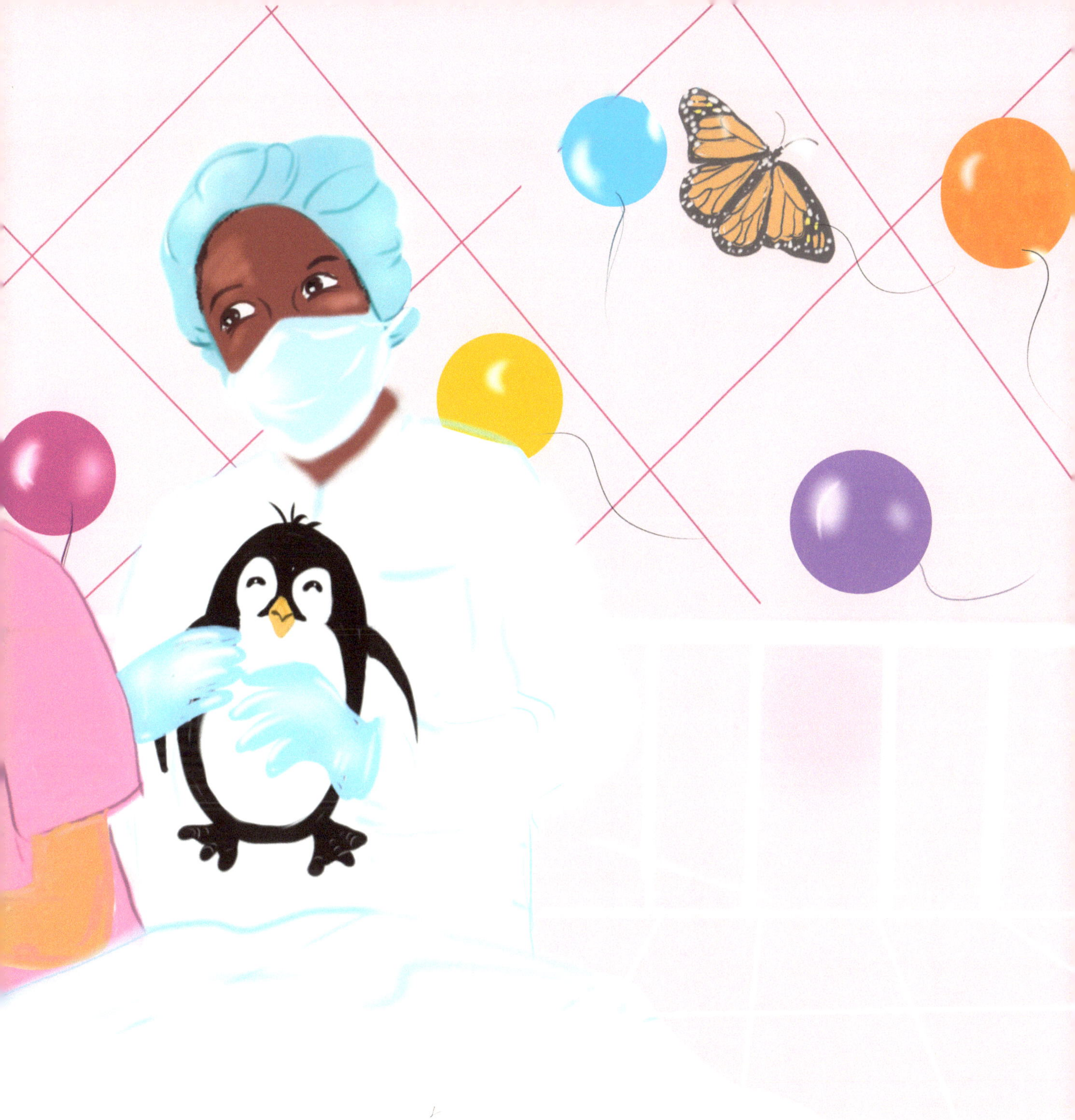

That is all I remember because I took a nap and dreamed while the doctors helped me.

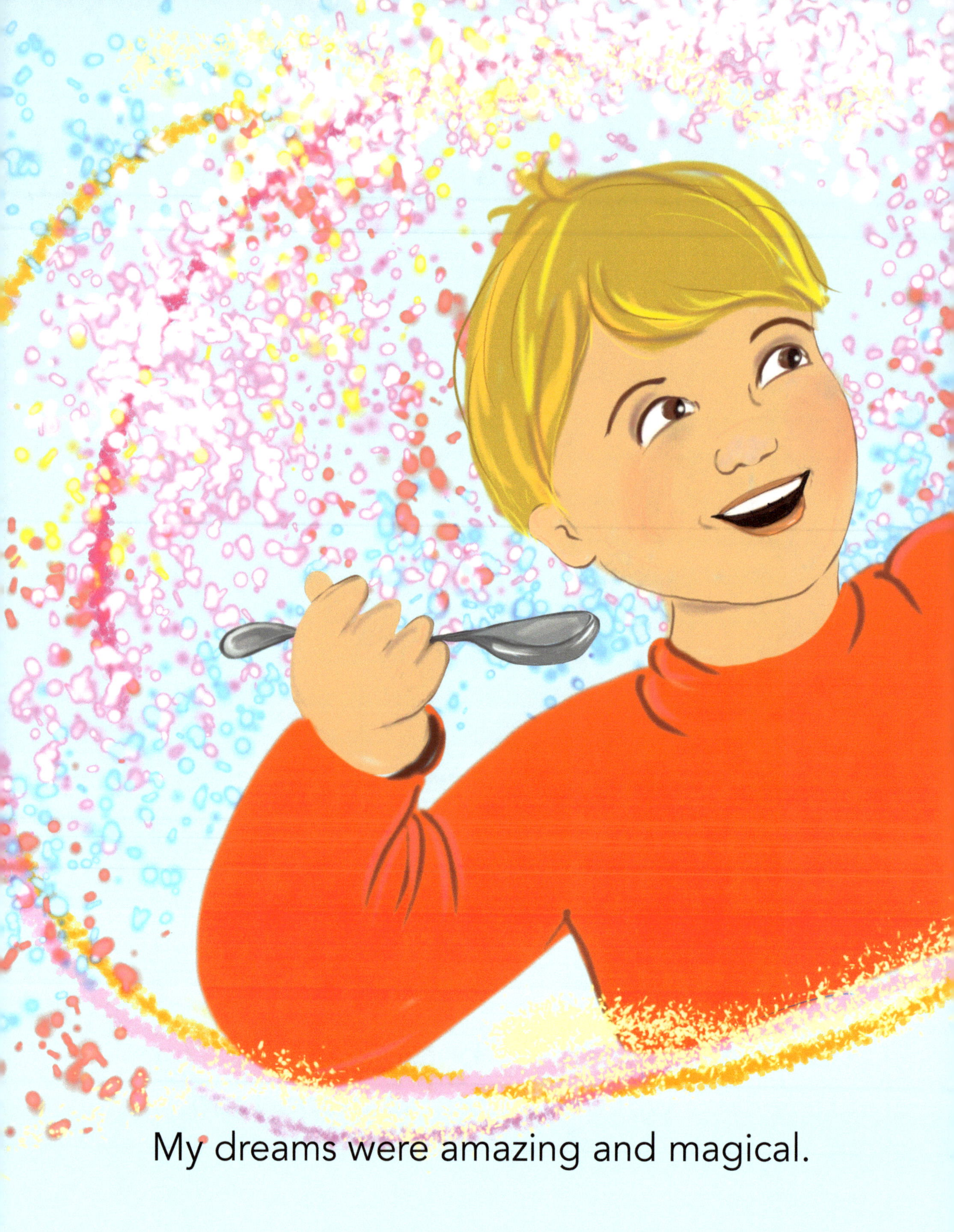

My dreams were amazing and magical.

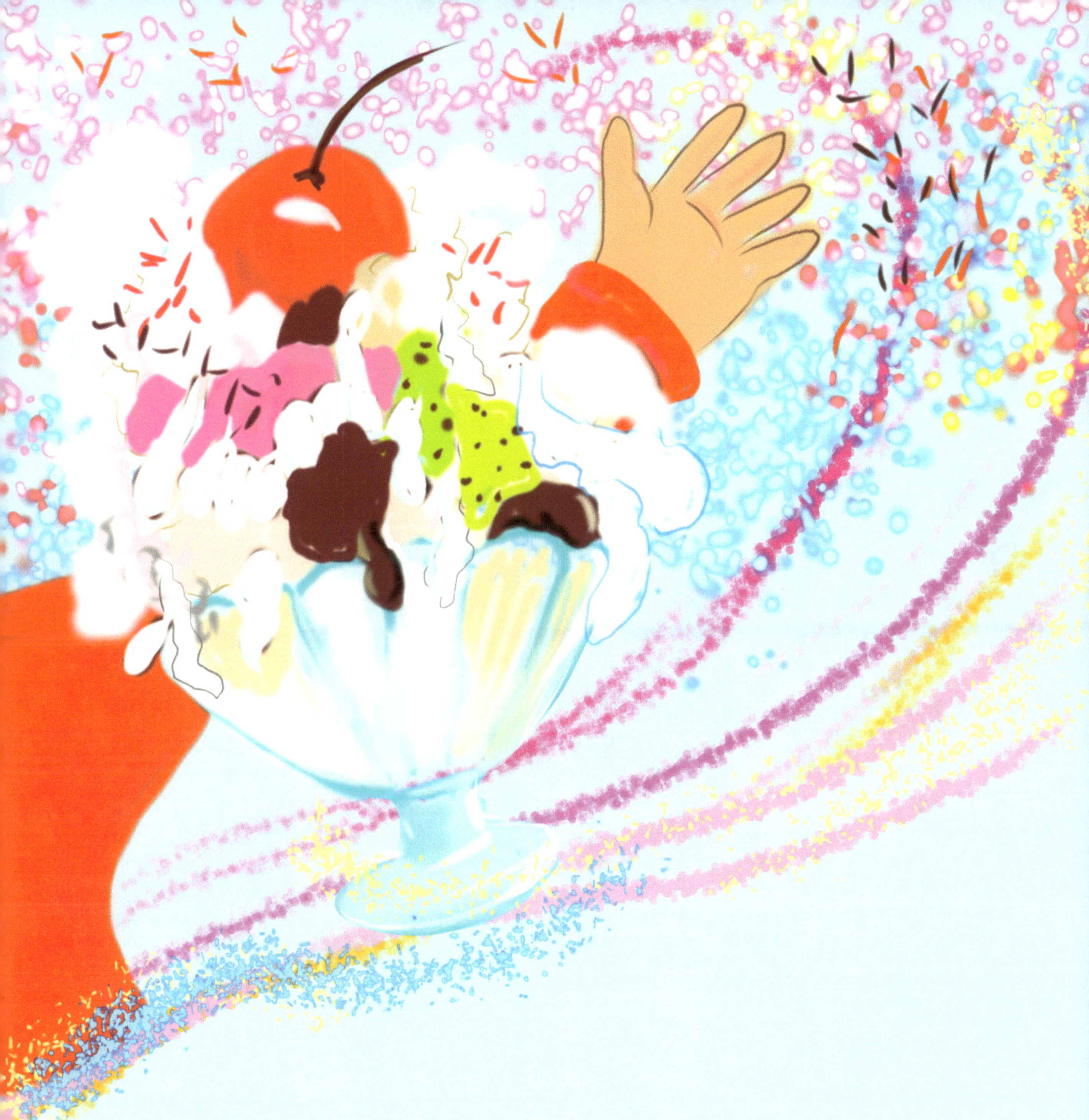

I dreamed of a gigantic ice cream sundae with gooey marshmallow sauce, whipped cream, and the biggest cherry one has ever seen. Yum!

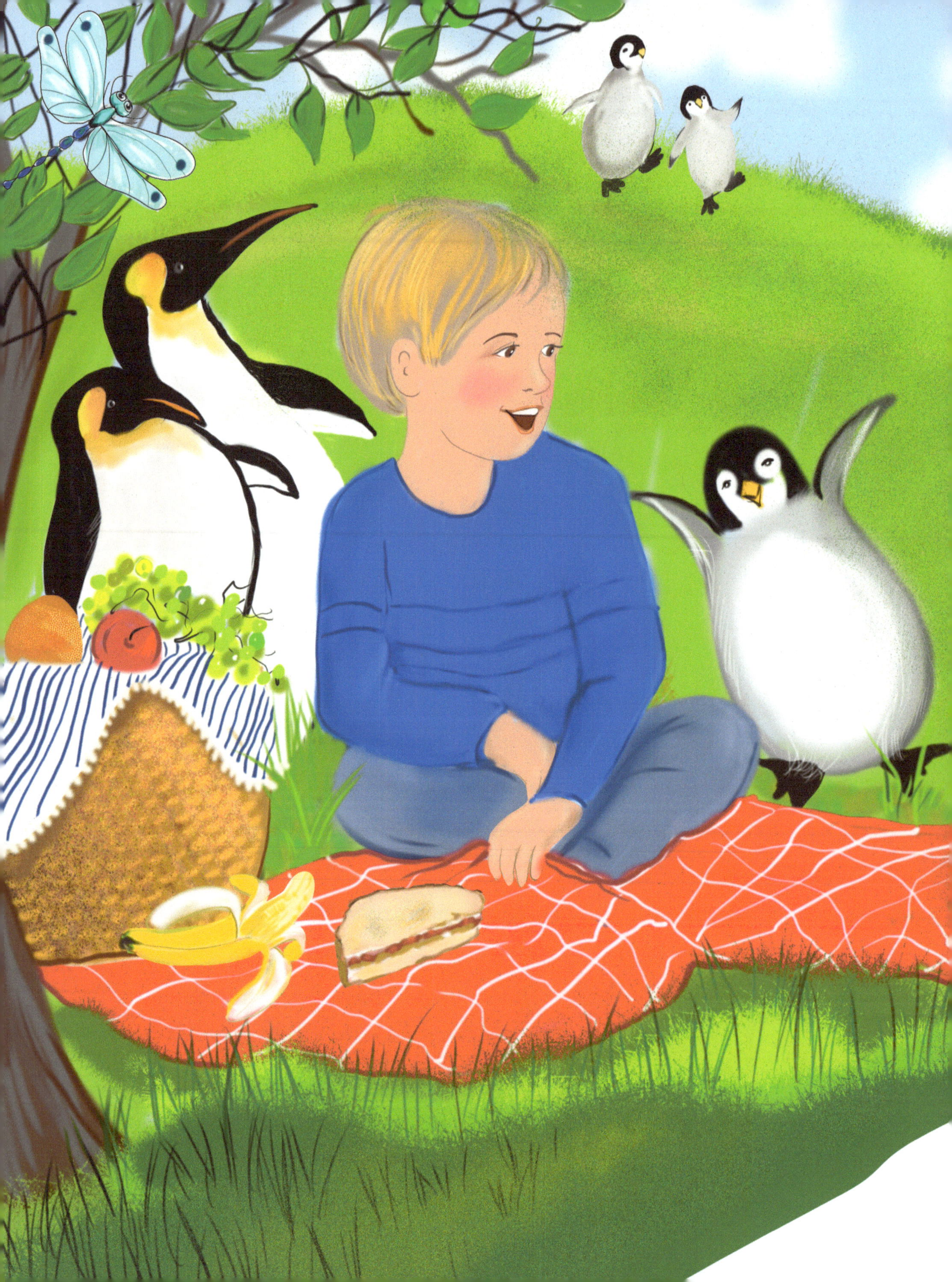

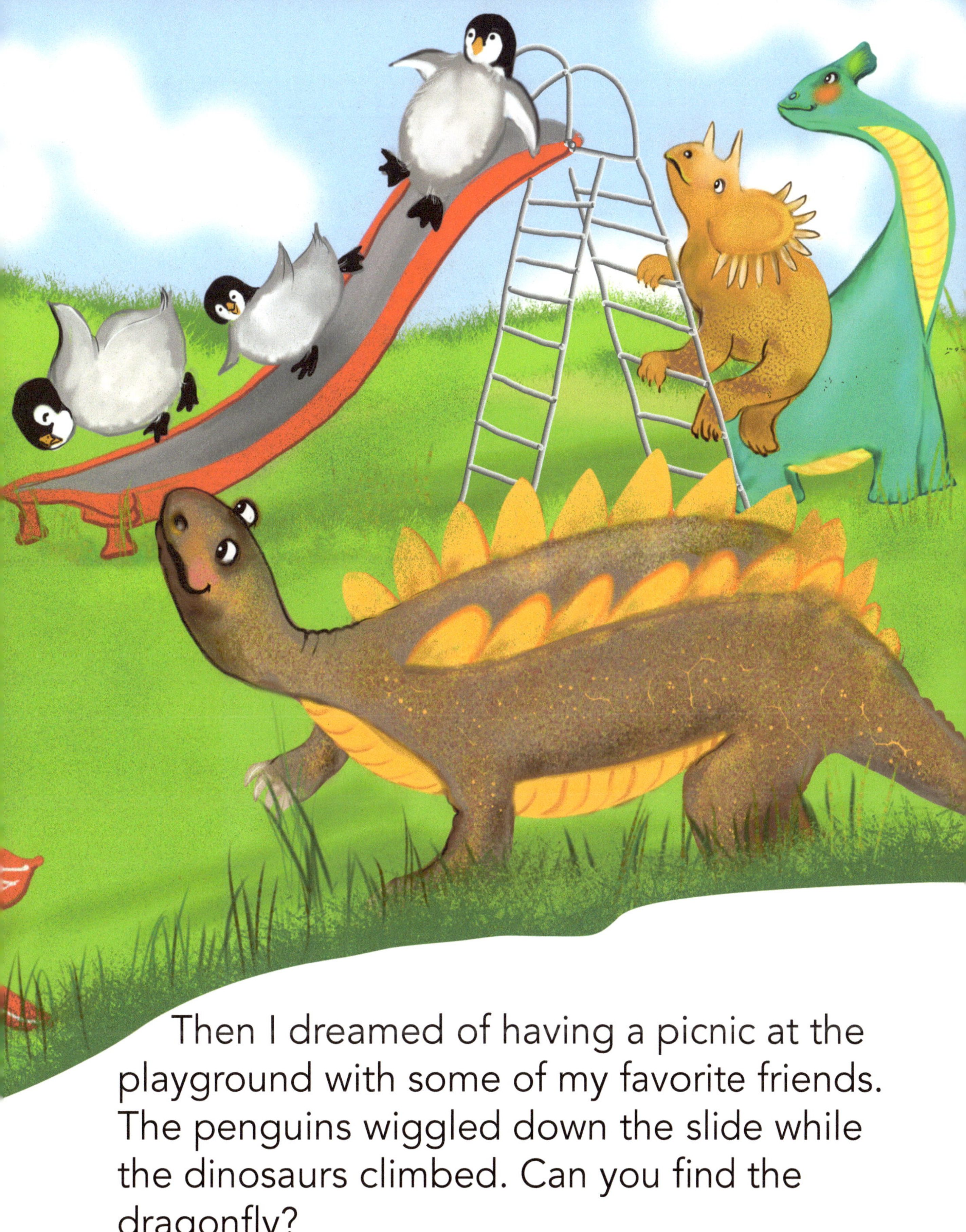

Then I dreamed of having a picnic at the playground with some of my favorite friends. The penguins wiggled down the slide while the dinosaurs climbed. Can you find the dragonfly?

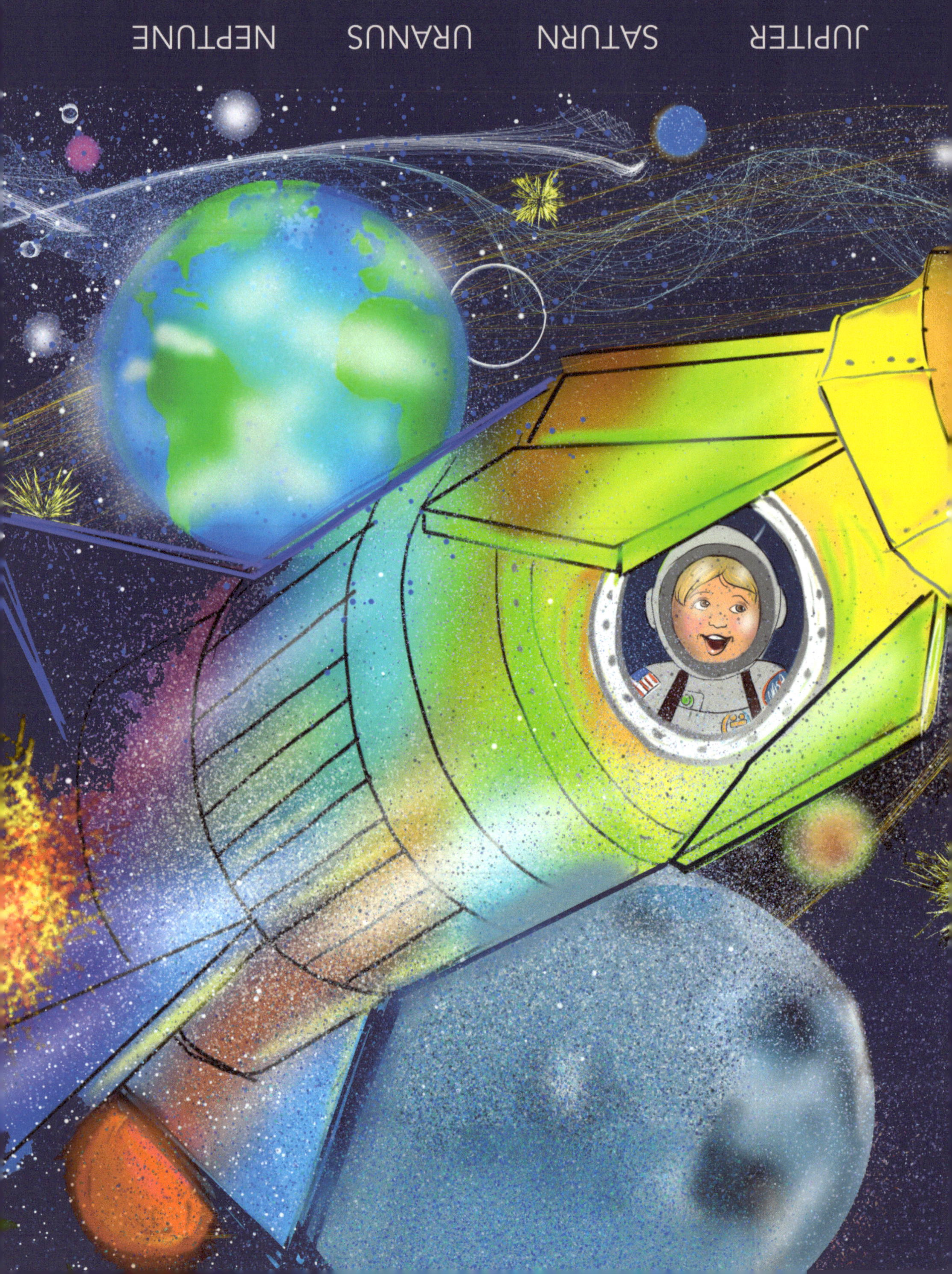
JUPITER
SATURN
URANUS
NEPTUNE

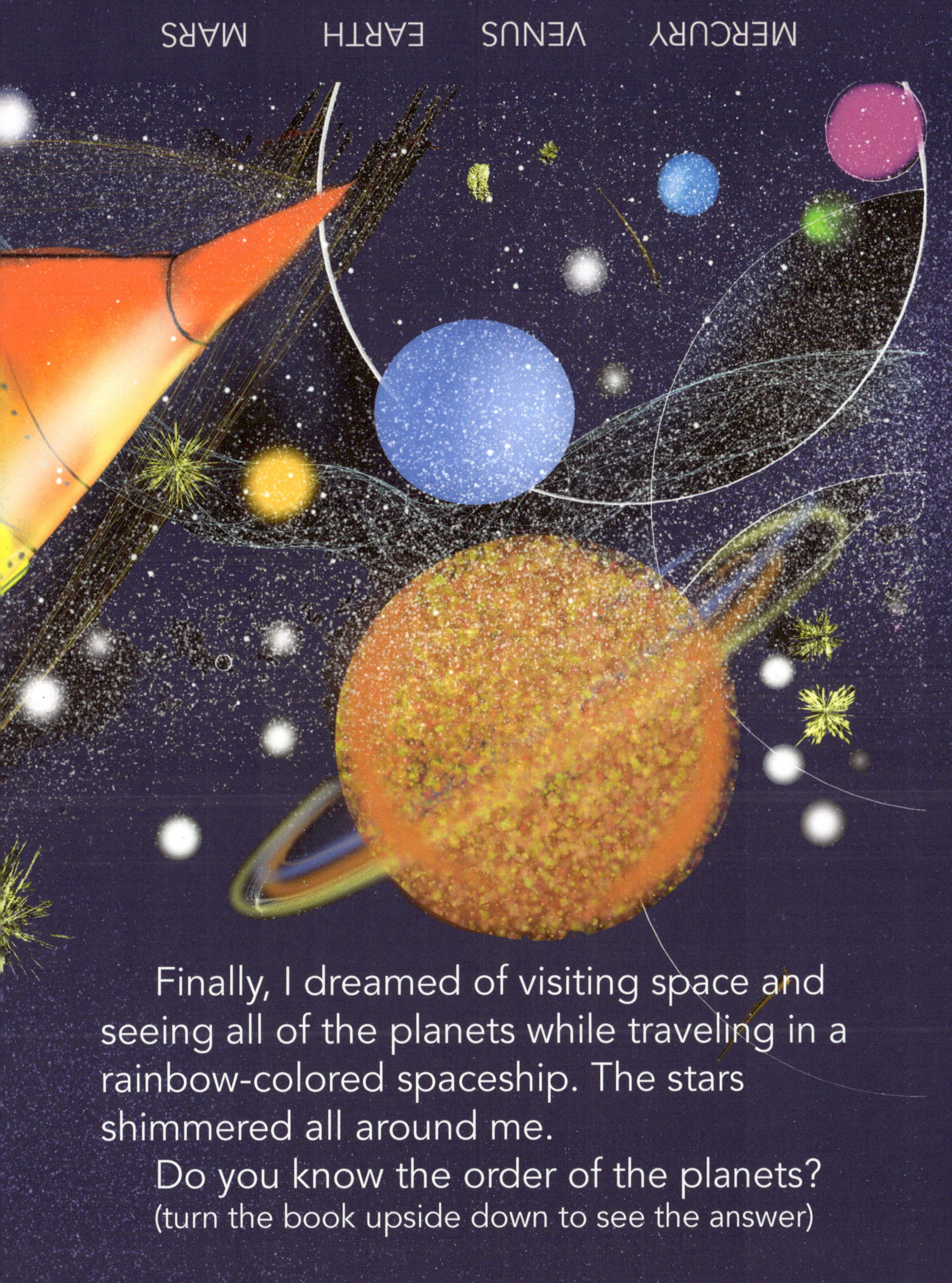

MARS    EARTH    VENUS    MERCURY
Finally, I dreamed of visiting space and seeing all of the planets while traveling in a rainbow-colored spaceship. The stars shimmered all around me.
Do you know the order of the planets?
(turn the book upside down to see the answer)

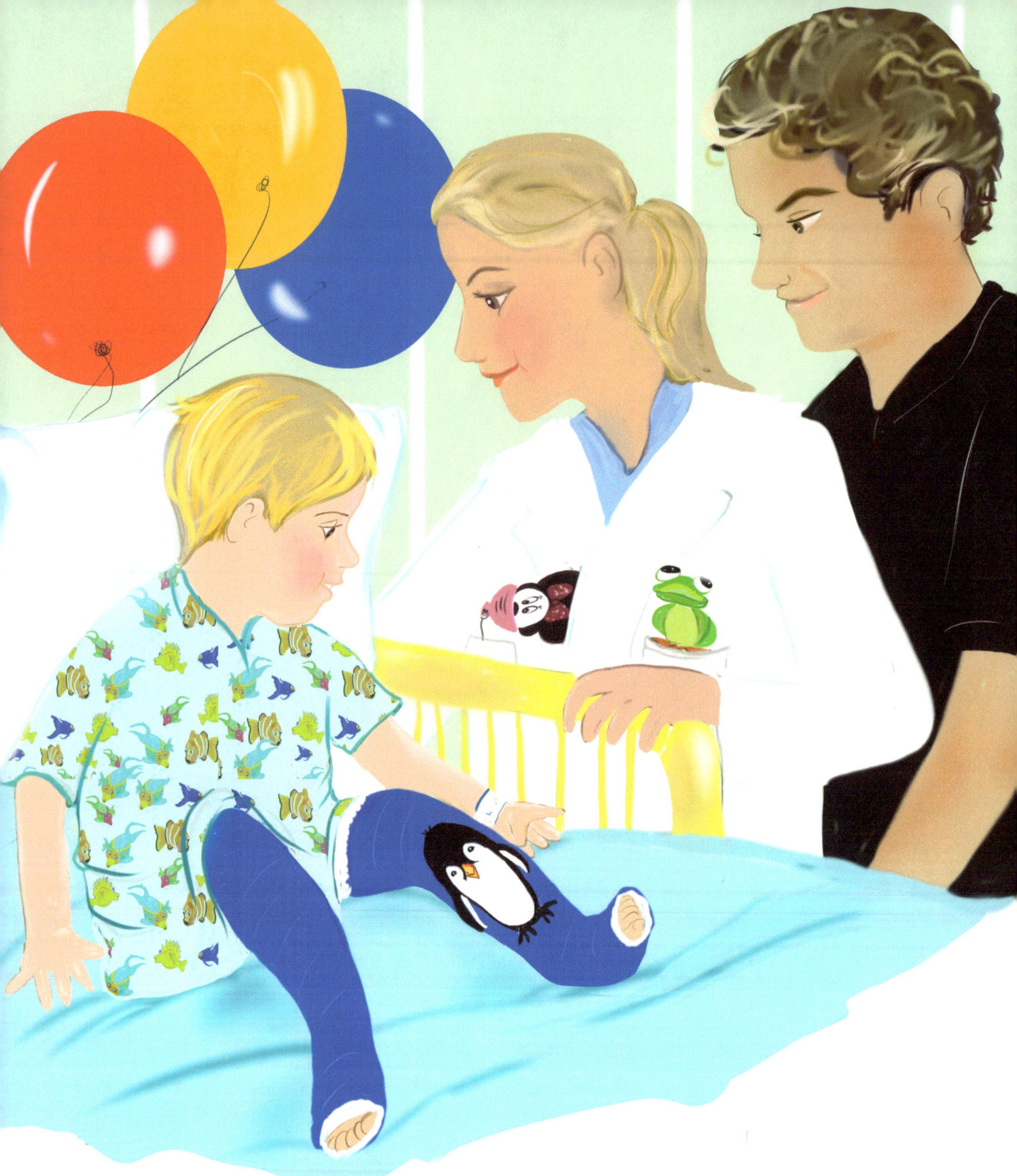

I awoke to see my wish came true. See the penguin on my blue cast!

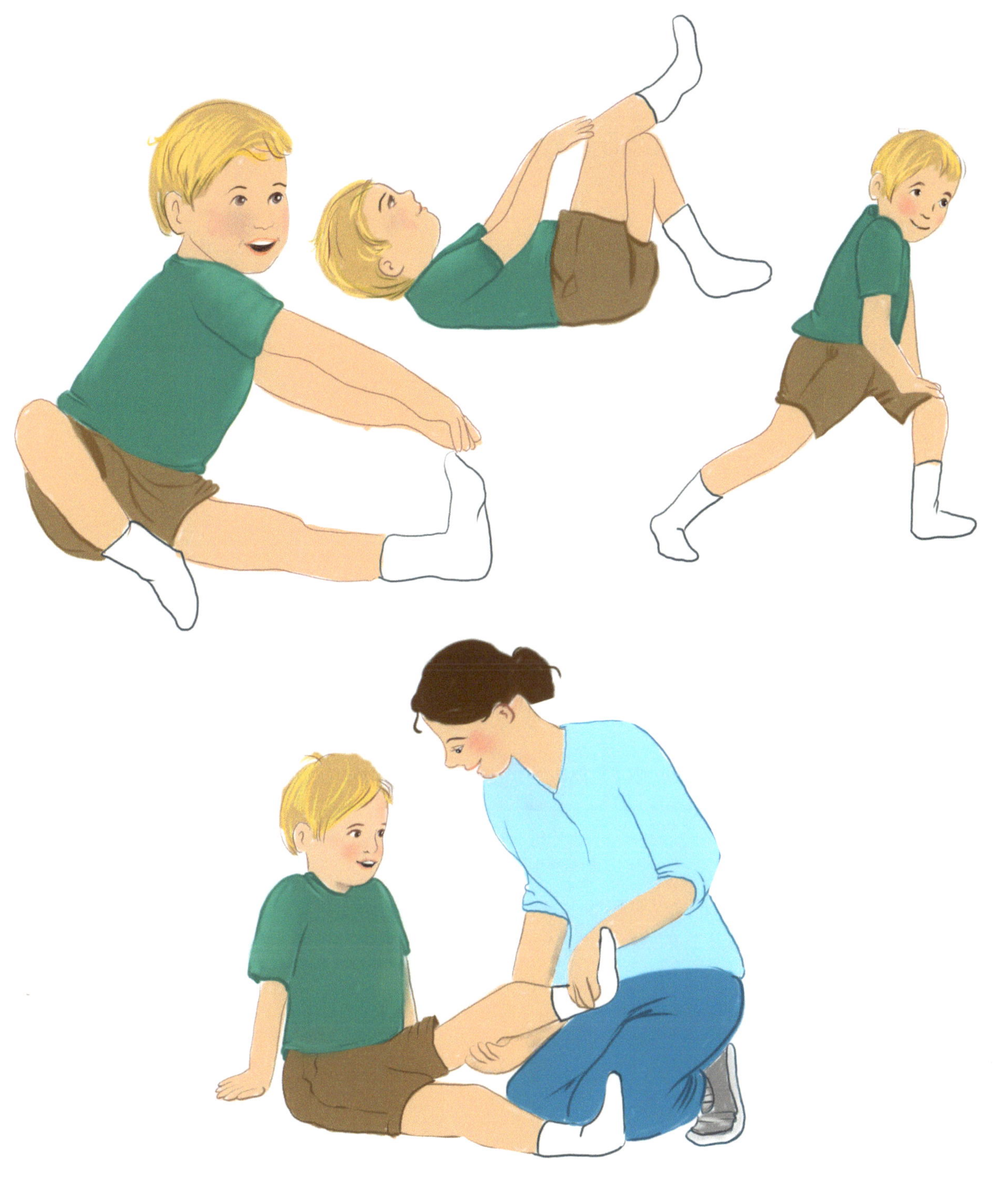

I had casts after surgery for about six weeks. I had so much fun with physical therapy. These are the doctors that help make you stronger over time.

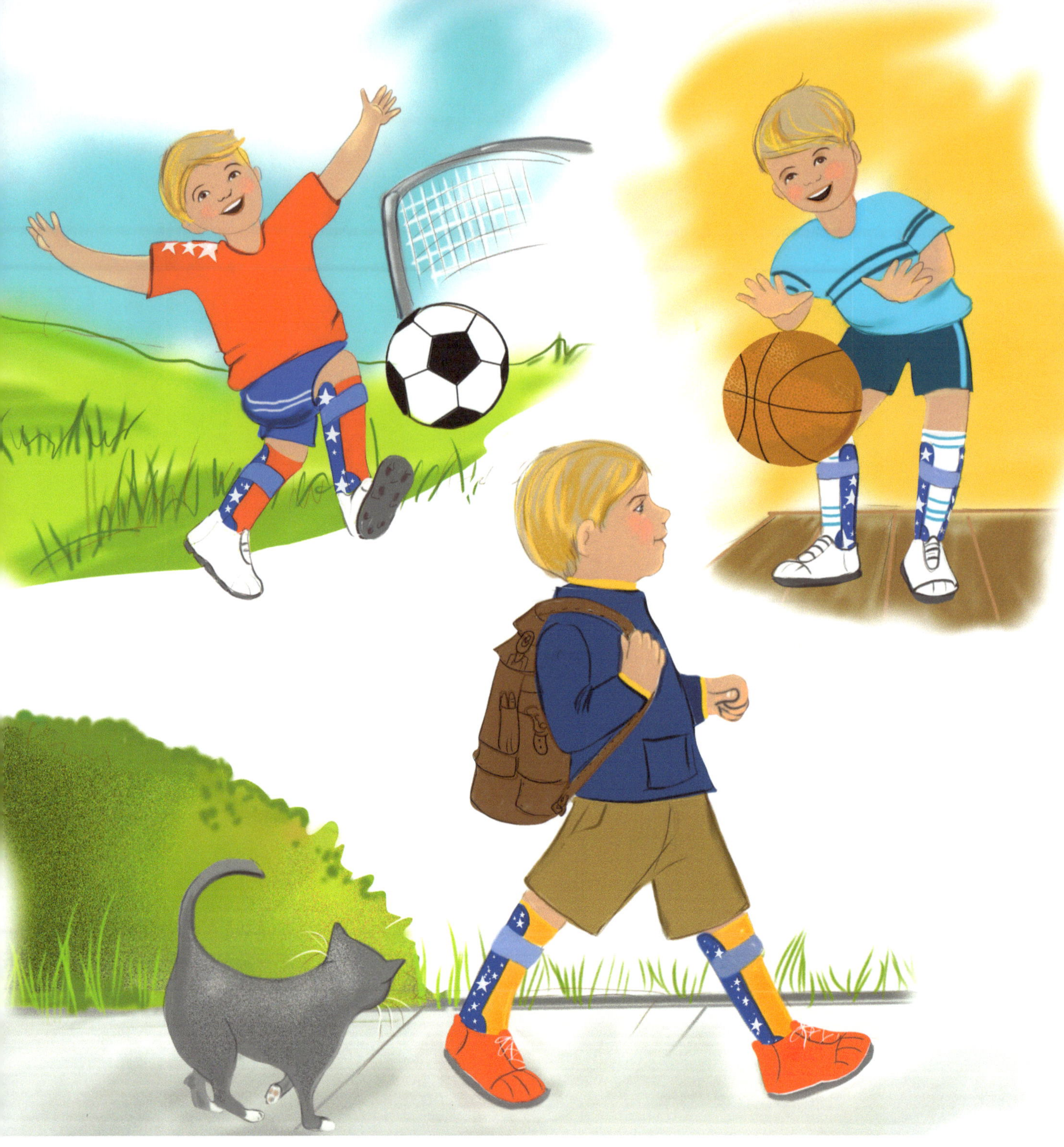

I now have braces to help me walk while I get stronger. Wearing my braces help keep my feet straight. I call them my big boots. There are many reasons children may need braces.

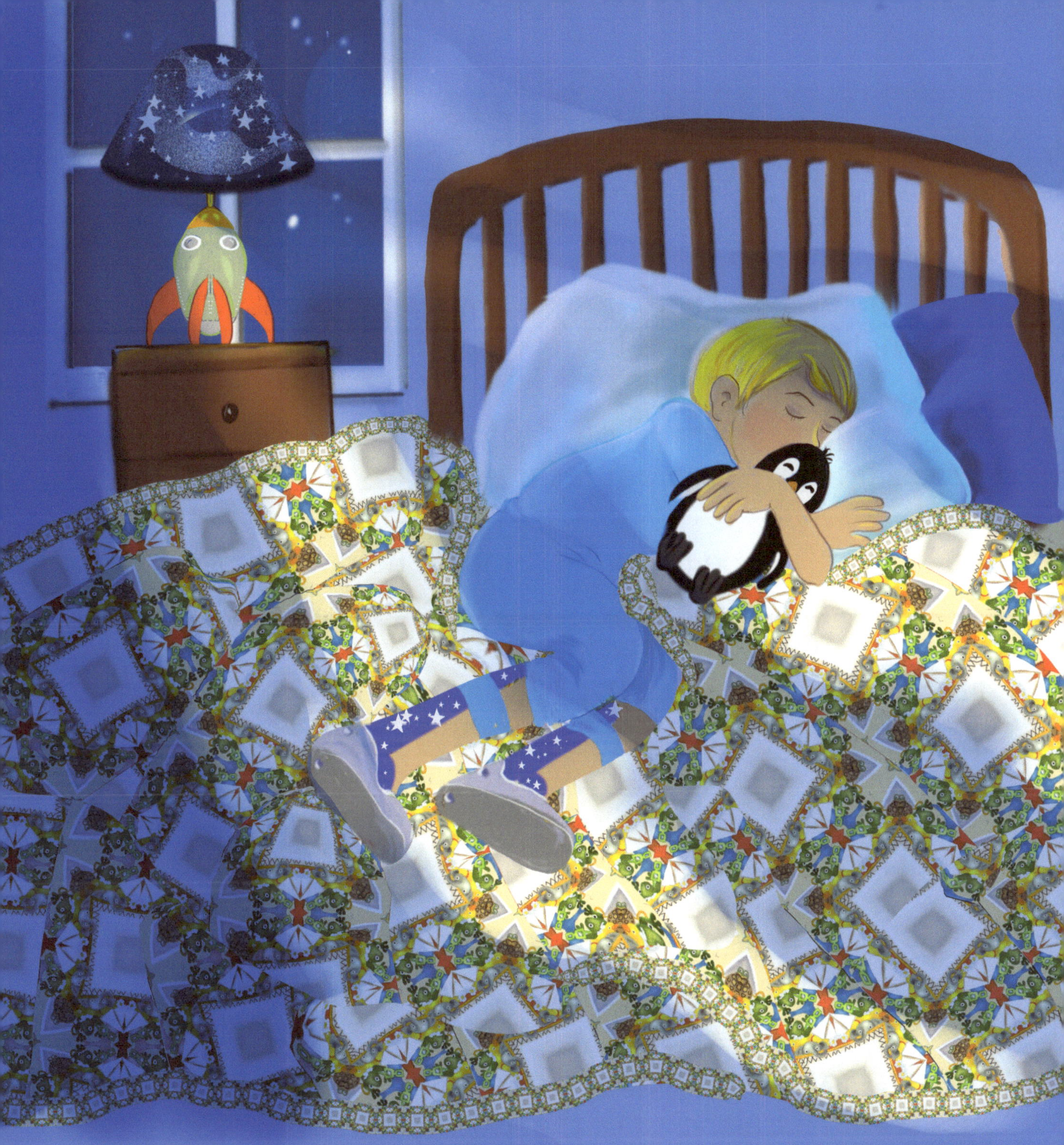

Some children wear braces all day and all night. My big boots provide a stretch at night while I am sleeping.

# Fun Facts

• The Ponseti Method contains a series of maneuvers to manipulate the foot into an improved position.
Well-molded casts are generally changed weekly.
The method is utilized to treat clubfoot and recurrences.

• Bracing discontinued prior to the age of four has been associated with clubfoot recurrence.

• Clubfoot can be recurrent. Bracing helps minimize recurrence while some children will still develop return of clubfoot features. It is important to maintain close follow up with the child's physician.

• Clubfoot recurrences may not fully be corrected with casting alone. Some children need surgical procedures to rebalance the foot.

• Typical soft tissue procedures include lengthening or release of the Achilles to reduce tightness in the back of the leg. Some children benefit from a Tibialis Anterior Tendon transfer to minimize clubfoot recurrences and assist with rebalancing of the foot. Other tendons can also be transferred or released.

• Older children with rigid deformities may require bone procedures to realign the foot. Wires and/or hardware may be utilized to promote bone healing and stabilization.

• Often casts are utilized leading into surgery and children are casted following surgery. Time frames depend on procedures performed.  Bracing may be utilized after surgery to maintain correction, to provide stability, and/or  to stretch muscle groups that have a tendency to tighten. Bracing may be temporary or lifelong based on the child's needs.

• Some children with neurologic and/or motor weakness may require specific daytime bracing to promote stability and function along with nighttime bracing to minimize contractures and recurrence.

• ADMs may be used in the setting of neuromuscular conditions with hip and/or knee contractures. Research is ongoing for use in younger patients.

 For more information please visit: **drmitziwilliams.com, dobbsclubfoot.com, dobbsbrace.com, and kiddfoot.com**

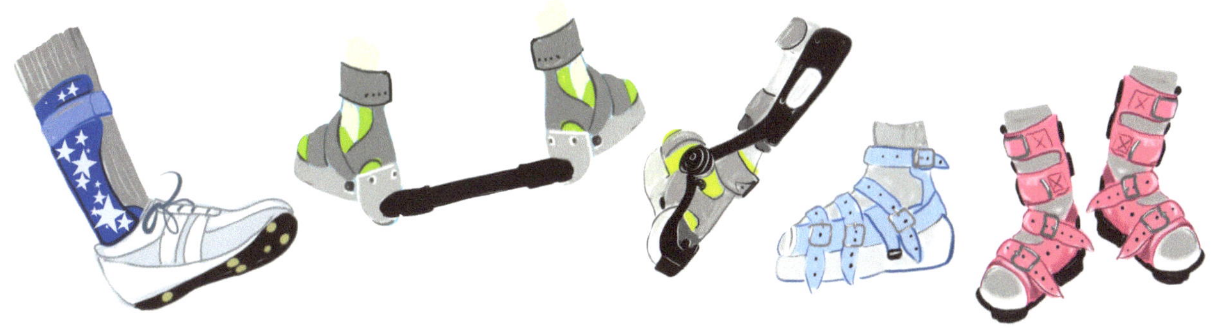

# Draw and color your own cast!

# Here are some of our favorite casts!
## Circle the one <u>you</u> like the best.

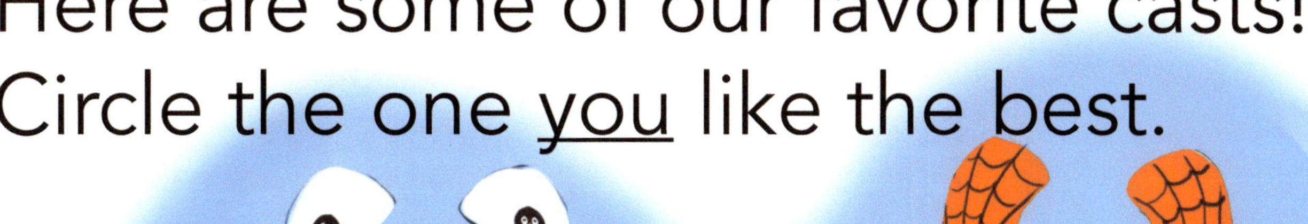

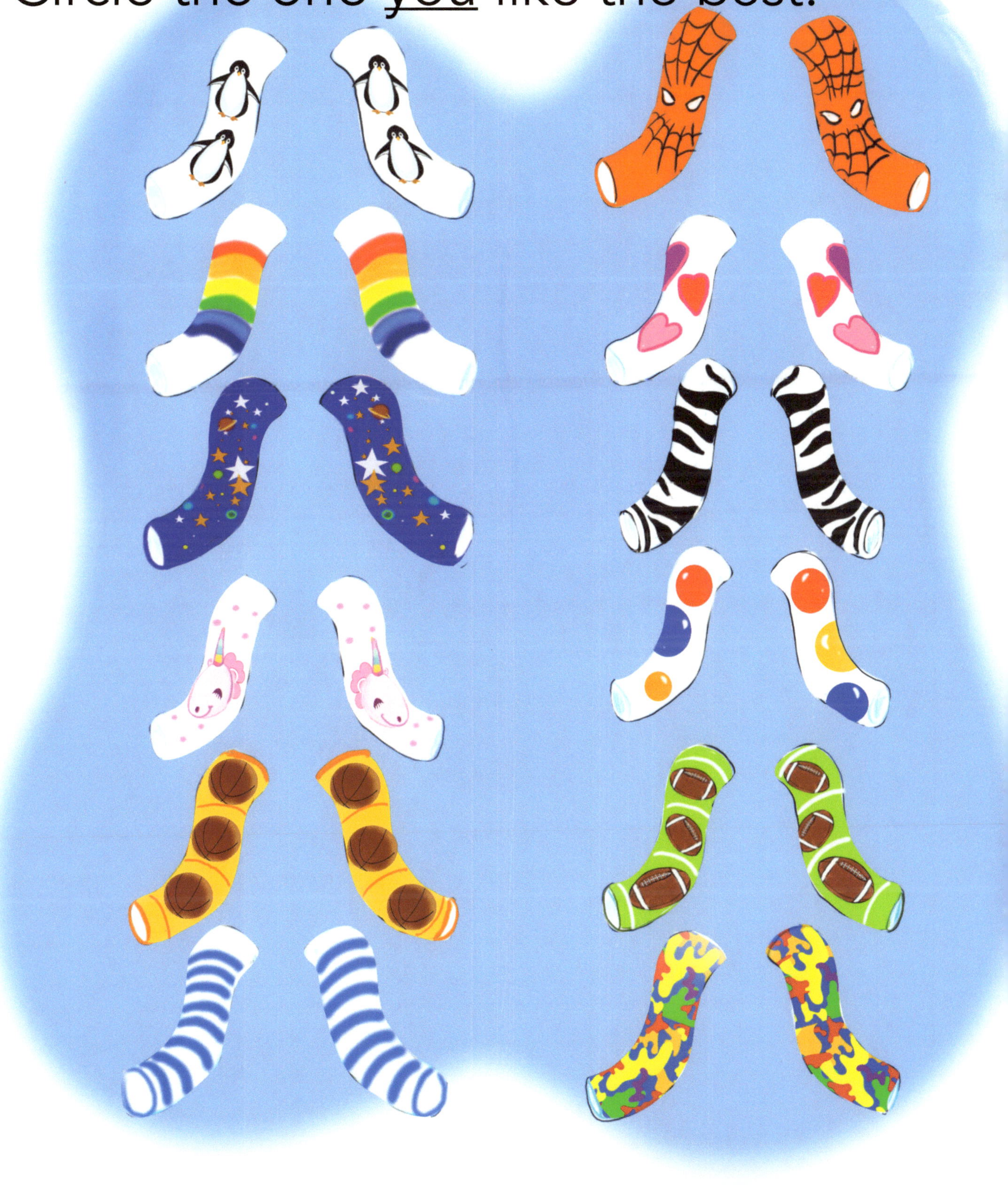